The Drug Conversation: How to Talk to Your Child about Drugs

Dr Owen Bowden-Jones

RCPsych Publications

RCPsych Publications is an imprint of the Royal College of Psychiatrists,
21 Prescot Street, London E1 8BB
http://www.rcpsych.ac.uk

British Library Cataloguing-in-Publication Data.
A catalogue record for this book is available from the British Library.
ISBN 978-1-909726-57-4

Distributed in North America by Publishers Storage and Shipping Company.

The views presented in this book do not necessarily reflect those of the Royal College of Psychiatrists, and the publishers are not responsible for any error of omission or fact.

The Royal College of Psychiatrists is a charity registered in England and Wales (228636) and in Scotland (SC038369).

Printed in the UK by Latimer Trend and Company Ltd, Plymouth.

Contents

Acknowledgements

I would like to thank the following people for their support and advice in developing this book: Philippa, Rebecca, Anne-Catrin, Mo, David, Rachel, Tudor, Pat, Angelica, Francesca, Etta and the team at the Royal College of Psychiatrists, you have all been wonderful. Most of all, I am indebted to my patients and their families for sharing their journeys.

Introduction

'Mind your own business. What I do is up to me. You always go on about drugs being bad, but what do you know? You told me you've never taken any, right? So how do you know what's what? You don't know anything!' – a 15-year-old's response to being asked by his mother if he is taking drugs.

I'm sitting with Harry, a bright, articulate 15-year-old who attends a well-known school in London. Harry's parents are here too, looking anxious and frustrated. This is my second meeting with Harry and he is here because he uses drugs. He mostly uses cannabis but also occasionally ecstasy and, on one occasion, he has taken cocaine. To Harry's dismay, one of his friends told a teacher that they were worried about him. The head teacher called Harry and his parents to a meeting to discuss his progress and reported drug use.

Harry doesn't think his drug use is a problem, claiming that all of his friends smoke a joint (of cannabis) 'now and then' and that he uses less than some. Despite recently falling grades, Harry knows he is bright and wants to go to university to study journalism, something he has wanted to do for as long as he can remember. He seems relaxed, even confident, as he talks to me about how cannabis helps control his anxiety, improves his sleep and makes him feel relaxed and 'part of the crowd'. He can't imagine a life without drugs.

Harry's parents, on the other hand, are horrified. They can hardly bring themselves to believe that Harry is using drugs and blame his friends for introducing him to them. They think he has fallen in with a 'bad lot' and is putting his promising future at risk. At today's meeting, they ask Harry to stop using drugs immediately, threaten to ban him from seeing his friends and insist that he is drug-tested every week. They become frustrated and angry when he says that they are overreacting and accuses them of being out of touch and ignorant about drugs.

Tensions rise further as it becomes clear that Harry has been stealing money from his mother's purse to spend on cannabis. His parents also discover that at weekends he has repeatedly lied about where he is and whom he is with. The conversation becomes increasingly heated and hostile.

This story has unfolded hundreds of times in my office.

Months later, Harry has changed his mind. He found that his drug use started to affect important parts of his life. His academic performance dropped further and cannabis made him increasingly paranoid. With support, he has stopped using drugs completely, although he has not ruled out trying them again in the future. He has needed to change some of his friends but seems happier for this. The paranoia has improved and he is able to study again.

Harry's parents have also been working hard. They now know much more about drugs and what to look out for if Harry starts using again. They have had to learn to trust him again despite feeling anxious about this, but can see that Harry is making progress.

Unfortunately, not all stories end this well.

Why write this book?

I wrote this book for two reasons. The first is that I am a psychiatrist who specialises in drug problems. Over the years, I have met thousands of patients and helped them on their often complex and sometimes painful journey to recovery. As a psychiatrist, I am interested in both the brain systems underpinning drug misuse and the psychological reasons for these problems. I believe my patients and their families deserve clear and up-to-date information to help them make decisions. This book will give you plenty of information to help you understand how drugs affect the brain, what problems they cause and possible solutions.

The second reason for writing this book is that I am a parent. Like many parents, I worry about how I can best look after and support my children. Other parents clearly feel this too, and all ask me the same questions.

- How do I talk to my child about drugs?
- What should I look out for?
- Can I stop them from trying drugs?
- What should I do if I think they are using drugs?

Drug use arouses difficult feelings – confusion, anger, helplessness and condemnation. These feelings are understandable, but can sometimes make the situation worse.

In my experience, it is unhelpful to judge someone as 'bad' because they use drugs. It's far better to try to understand their reasons for using drugs. So, in this book I steer clear of moral judgements about drug use. There will always be people who want to experiment with drugs, but some people are damaged by these experiments. What I most want to do is to help people avoid this damage and to help those who have begun to experience harm, and their families, to find a better way to manage their lives.

Why read this book?

Most parents assume that their child will be taught about drugs by the school they attend. Many schools do a good job, but standards can vary. I always suggest that parents take an active role in educating their child about drugs, and don't rely entirely on schools.

Parents might worry about talking to their children about this subject and feel they don't have enough information to start a conversation about drugs. These concerns are understandable – the drug market is also very different now from when parents were growing up. There are now more drugs than ever, both illegal and legal. The internet is increasingly used to market and sell drugs.

This book will address all of these issues in a clear, practical way, focusing on what you need to know. Using the latest science, this book will help you feel more informed about drugs, more confident in talking to your child, more able to avoid problems developing and more prepared to tackle problems with drugs if they arise.

How to use this book

This book can be read in different ways. If you don't know much about drugs, then reading the chapters in order will give you the best introduction. However, all the chapters have been written to stand on their own, so you can go straight to the one that you need. So, if you have a particular question, such as 'How can I drug-test my child?' or 'I've just found drugs in their room, what should I do?' then you can skip to the relevant section. At the end of each section, there is a summary of the key points covered.

There are case studies from my clinical practice throughout the book that illustrate different points. All these patients consented to their stories being used, but names and other details have been changed to ensure anonymity.

What are psychoactive drugs, who uses them and why?

What are psychoactive drugs?

A psychoactive drug is a chemical substance that alters the functioning of the brain, causing changes in the way we think, feel and behave. All drugs can be divided into those that have psychoactive effects and those that don't. Most drugs, for example medications like antibiotics, are not psychoactive. Antibiotics treat infections but they don't change our emotions.

Psychoactive drugs can be stimulating, sedating, cause hallucinations or produce an out-of-body state called dissociation. Some psychoactive drugs can cause more than one of these effects.

How much of a problem are psychoactive drugs?

Before we talk more about psychoactive drugs and the problems they can cause, let's look at how commonly they are used. The United Nations Office on Drugs and Crime (2014) estimates that around one person in twenty of the world's population between 15 and 64 years of age has used an illicit psychoactive drug in the past year. That's around 250 million people. Of these people, about one in ten experience problems with their drug use. The same report estimates that, globally, 183 000 people a year die from drug-related causes: about 40 people per million.

The UK government conducts an annual survey estimating drug misuse in England and Wales (Home Office, 2014). It shows that around one in three adults have taken an illicit drug at some point during their lives, and about one in twelve have used drugs in the past year. As with all surveys, some people will not tell the truth, inflating or reducing the estimates, but a yearly survey does give an indication of changes in patterns of drug use over time. The survey results suggest that the past decade has seen a gradual reduction in the number of people using drugs, and this seems to be true for all age groups.

While heroin use seems to be declining in the general population and in young people in particular, other drugs seem to be gaining popularity: cannabis and the so-called legal highs. Most newer drugs are not accurately recorded in surveys, so their use is likely to be underestimated. Chapter 6 discusses them in more detail.

Young people and drug use

Psychoactive drug use is more common in younger people. Many young people who use psychoactive drugs will do so briefly (perhaps out of curiosity), decide it is not for them and stop. A small proportion of users, however, will begin to use more regularly. In general, the more often a psychoactive drug is used, the greater the likelihood that it will cause problems.

So what does the UK survey tell us about young people? Looking at those between 16 and 24 years of age, more than one in three have used a psychoactive drug at some point in their lives, equivalent to around 2.2 million people. One in five young people used drugs in the past year (Home Office, 2014).

When do young people start using drugs?

The UK government also measures drug use in school-aged children. Around a quarter of 15-year-olds report having taken a drug at some point in their lives, and a fifth reported use in the past year (Health and Social Care Information Centre, 2015). A quarter of children 11–15 years of age had been offered a drug, even if they chose not to take it.

Another estimate of drug use in young people comes from the USA. The Monitoring the Future project (www.monitoringthefuture.org) has recorded drug use in US school-aged children since 1975. Approximately 50 000 pupils take part in the annual survey and, like the annual survey of England and Wales, it can track trends over time. The US survey suggests even higher levels of drug use. More than a third of US 15-year-olds report drug use at some point; over a quarter in the past year.

Both the UK and US figures suggest that many young people have experimented with drugs by their mid-teens. This is important when we think about the best time to start talking to our children about psychoactive drugs.

Which drugs are young people using?

The popularity of different drugs changes over time and with user age. Fig. 1.1 shows the patterns of drug use by UK schoolchildren. The use of volatile substances such as glue peaks at around 13 or 14 years old before declining. Cannabis use, however, takes off at that age, with a fivefold increase between 13 and 15 years of age.

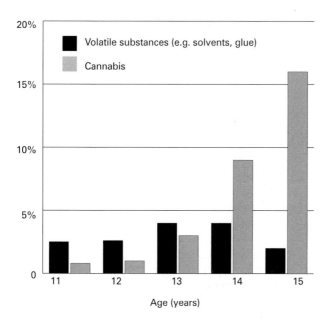

Fig. 1.1 Percentage of children 11–16 years of age who have taken volatile substances and cannabis in the past year, by age. Adapted from Health and Social Care Information Centre (2015).

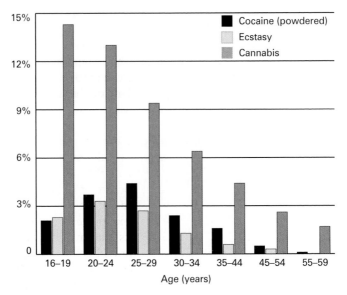

Fig. 1.2 Percentage of people 16–59 years of age who have used cocaine, ecstasy or cannabis in the past year, by age. Source: Home Office (2014).

From 16 years of age onwards, cannabis remains the most common drug across all age groups but peaks in the late teens (Fig. 1.2). Ecstasy (3,4-methylenedioxymethamphetamine, or MDMA) use peaks in the early 20s and powder cocaine use is most common in the late 20s.

Drug preference is influenced by many factors, including availability, cost and perceived acceptability. Some drugs are associated with particular social or ethnic groups. For example, the electronic dance music scene is associated with the stimulant drug ecstasy (Winstock *et al*, 2001).

What do young people think about drugs?

Most adolescents disapprove of using psychoactive drugs. Asked the question 'Is it OK to try taking cannabis to see what it is like?', less than one in twenty UK children under 13 years of age agreed. But by 15 years of age, one in five answered yes. At this age, trying cannabis was still less acceptable than trying tobacco (half of all 15-year-olds agree) or alcohol (three-quarters of 15-year-olds agree) (Health and Social Care Information Centre, 2014).

The Monitoring the Future project also asks school-aged US children about attitudes. Rather than asking if drug use is acceptable, they ask if the children disapprove of different drugs. By 15–16 years of age, only half of the US children surveyed disapproved of cannabis. Disapproval of other drugs remained high (Miech *et al*, 2015).

Although we can't directly compare the UK and US results – because they ask different questions – the overall findings are strikingly similar. Most children in their early to mid-teens disapprove of drugs, but drugs become more acceptable as they get older. Why do their attitudes change? In general, attitudes change because of new information and the opinions of those around you. As adolescents mature and explore their expanding worlds, what they are told about drugs, and by whom, is likely to be very influential. Having the right information is important at any age, but for adolescents having the right information is essential.

What about the law?

Many psychoactive drugs, such as heroin or cocaine, are illegal because of their harmful effects on the user. The legal status of a particular drug differs from country to country, but in general, drugs that cause more harm have stricter controls. In the UK, illegal drugs are divided into three broad categories: Class A, Class B and Class C. These classes carry different penalties for producing, selling or possessing (Table 1.1).

Key messages

- Drug use is common. It is estimated that a third of people in the UK have tried a psychoactive drug.
- Young people use more drugs than any other age group, many by their mid-teens.
- Cannabis is the most commonly used psychoactive drug (excluding alcohol).

Table 1.1   UK drug classes and maximum penalties for possession and supply/production

Class	Drug	Maximum penalty for possession	Maximum penalty for supply and production
A	Crack cocaine, cocaine, ecstasy, heroin, lysergic acid diethylamide (LSD), magic mushrooms, methadone, methamphetamine (crystal meth)	Up to 7 years in prison, an unlimited fine, or both	Up to life in prison, an unlimited fine, or both
B	Amphetamines, barbiturates, cannabis, codeine, ketamine, methylphenidate (Ritalin®), synthetic cannabinoids, synthetic cathinones (e.g. mephedrone, methoxetamine)	Up to 5 years in prison, an unlimited fine, or both	Up to life in prison, an unlimited fine, or both
C	Anabolic sterioids, benzodiazepines (diazepam), gamma-hydroxybutyrate (GHB), gamma-butyrolactone (GBL), piperazines (BZP), khat	Up to 2 years in prison, an unlimited fine, or both (except anabolic steroids – it's not an offence to possess them for personal use)	Up to 14 years in prison, an unlimited fine, or both
Temporary class[a]		None, but police can take away a suspected temporary class drug	Up to 14 years in prison, an unlimited fine, or both

a. The government can ban new drugs for 1 year under a temporary banning order while they decide how the drugs should be classified. Source: www.gov.uk/penalties-drug-possession-dealing.

What about alcohol?

This book looks at psychoactive drugs, but not alcohol. This does not mean that alcohol is not a psychoactive drug – it is. In fact, it is the most commonly consumed psychoactive drug in many countries. Alcohol accounts for around 6% of all deaths globally. Although it can be used without harm to the individual, it also creates significant and widespread damage. According to the World Health Organization (2014), around 16% of the world's population engages in heavy episodic drinking, with wealthy countries generally consuming more alcohol per person. However, many parents will be far more knowledgeable about alcohol than psychoactive drugs and it is this knowledge gap that this book is designed to fill in. Having said this, many of the approaches described in this book can also be used with problem drinking.

Why do people use drugs?

People take drugs to change the way they feel, even if only for a short time. Psychoactive drugs are a powerful and reliable way to change a person's psychological state. They can be stimulating (making the user feel energised), sedating (leading to feelings of calm and relaxation), hallucinogenic (causing vivid perceptual changes) or dissociative (resulting in 'out-of-body' or 'near-death' experiences). Most drugs work quickly, are relatively cheap and widely available. Some of my patients tell me that if they wanted to, they could buy drugs within 20 minutes of leaving my office. So, if you want to use a psychoactive drug, it's easy to find it.

If we accept that using a psychoactive drug is a reliable, if potentially high-risk, way to change the way you feel, then the question becomes why do people want to feel different in the first place? Psychoactive drugs affect the brain by either giving a person new feelings or taking away existing feelings. In essence, people take drugs to feel good, or to stop feeling bad.

Drugs to give new feelings or to numb existing feelings

Here are two very different scenarios.

John's story

John is 16 years old. He is going out clubbing with friends from school to celebrate the end of his summer exams. He has been looking forward to it all week and knows that the party will begin on Friday evening and continue all night. He is going to a new club and is really excited about the DJs and venue. John and his friends plan to take drugs, in this case the stimulant drug ecstasy. A few days ago they bought enough pills for all of them from a friend of a friend.

On Friday, John meets his friends at a bar and they have a few drinks before heading to the club. John is feeling in the mood to celebrate but also feels physically tired from late nights spent studying. They reach the club around 11 pm and once inside they all take their first dose of ecstasy.

Within about half an hour, the drug takes effect. John is now excited, full of energy and very sociable. He's aware that he is talking too much and can't keep still. He can't stop himself from grinning – a well-known side-effect of ecstasy. The music and lasers become more intense as the ecstasy takes effect. As he dances, John experiences an intense, overpowering euphoria. He describes feeling 'higher than heaven'.

Around 2 am, John begins to flag as his energy levels drop. It is time for another dose. John is an experienced ecstasy user and has judged from the effects of the first pill that this ecstasy is probably stronger than he is used to. He also knows that the more he takes, the greater the 'crash' will be over the next few days, so decides to take half a tablet and 'play it safe'.

The second dose works quickly and soon John is back dancing with his friends and really enjoying himself. Towards the end of the night, about 5.30 am, the second dose begins to wear off. John doesn't want to use any more ecstasy as he has plans to meet a friend on Sunday and doesn't want to spend his weekend recovering from the drug's effects. Instead he moves to the club's chill-out room to cool down. His friends agree that the night has been a spectacular success and that the DJs were brilliant.

John and his friends leave the club about 7 am on Saturday morning feeling physically tired but still mentally very alert from the ecstasy. They know they won't be able to sleep yet, so they all go and have breakfast before heading home. John arrives at his friend's house around 10 am, still feeling 'wired'. He smokes half a joint of cannabis to calm himself and eventually falls asleep around 11 am.

Over the next few days, John feels flat and exhausted. His concentration is poor and he is more irritable than usual. He is well aware that these are the effects of his ecstasy use, as he has experienced them many times before. The feelings peak on Monday afternoon when, for a few hours, John feels sad and upset, but he knows these feelings will pass and believes it is a price worth paying for his night out with friends.

By Thursday, he is feeling back to normal. John makes a mental note to not use ecstasy for the next couple of weeks to give his brain 'a rest' but later that day a friend messages him, inviting him to a new club the following evening. It sounds like it will be an amazing evening, and John starts to think it might be too good to miss.

John, an experienced ecstasy user, takes the drug to give him feelings that he would otherwise struggle to achieve or maintain. He carefully plans his use of ecstasy to give him the maximum benefit while minimising the negative effects. He also uses the sedative effects of cannabis to calm himself down and help him sleep.

His story is typical of many recreational drug users, who think carefully about the dose they want to use and often combine more than one drug to achieve the best effect. Mixing a stimulant and sedative drug is particularly common – ecstasy and cannabis or cocaine and alcohol are good examples. Whether John has as much control over his drug use as he thinks is unclear.

Jake's story

Jake has worked in the customer service department of a large company since leaving school a year ago. He is a studious, precise and shy person who describes himself as 'always a bit nervous around people'. Jake likes his job and is good at it. He was recently promoted and now manages a team of 14 people. Since his promotion, Jake has felt much more pressure due to the increased responsibility of managing his team but also from his new boss to hit company performance targets. He has found the work increasingly challenging and returns home from work most days feeling stressed, worried that he is not up to the job and that he will end up being demoted or sacked.

Jake has never really been interested in drugs, with the exception of cannabis, which he has used on and off since he was 14 years old. He now buys small amounts from a friend and smokes it on his own in his flat a few times a week as a 'bit of a treat'. It helps him relax, particularly after stressful days at work.

Over the past 6 months, Jake has noticed that his cannabis use has gradually increased and that he is now smoking every evening. In fact, over the past few weeks, the first thing he does when he gets home from work is smoke a joint, later followed by two more joints before he goes to sleep. He now finds that without cannabis, he struggles to sleep and feels 'edgy'. Jake is worried about the cannabis use and blames work and his overbearing boss.

A few weeks ago, during a particularly difficult day at work when 5 of his 14 staff called in sick, Jake had a panic attack. He felt emotionally overwhelmed, distressed and paralysed by fear. Hyperventilating, and with his heart beating so fast he thought he was having a heart attack, Jake left the office and went outside for some air. All he could think about was that his boss was expecting him to report on the company performance targets that afternoon, targets Jake already knew had not been achieved.

Instead of going back to the office, he went home and rang a work colleague to explain that he was not feeling well. Once home, feeling very shaky and with his heart still racing, Jake rolled himself a large joint of cannabis, which he quickly smoked. Within a few minutes he felt himself calming down. He smoked a second then a third joint, by which time he was feeling much better. His anxiety had completely gone and was replaced by a powerful feeling of calm and well-being. Jake rolled a final joint before falling asleep.

The next day, even the prospect of going to work felt overwhelming to Jake, but he knew that his boss would be waiting for his presentation and would be angry if he did not show up. To calm himself, Jake smoked a 'small' joint of cannabis, just enough to reduce his anxiety until behind his desk. He rolled a second joint and put it in his wallet. Jake knew this was a risky thing to do, but couldn't think of any other way to cope.

A few weeks later, I met Jake at the clinic. He was in a terrible state, having been fired from work and overwhelmed with anxiety. He asked if I could help him. Although Jake felt cannabis was the main problem, it soon became clear that his anxiety was the main issue to tackle.

Jake uses cannabis to control his anxiety. He has probably always been more anxious than others and the sedating effects of cannabis, when used in moderation, have worked well for him over the years. But as his stress levels increased, so did his cannabis use. The recent panic attack made him fearful of losing control at work.

Unfortunately for Jake, the more frequently cannabis is smoked, the greater the risk of tolerance. Tolerance develops when the brain becomes used to a drug through repeated consumption. The brain's receptors adjust to repeated drug use by making themselves less sensitive to the drug. Therefore, the user needs to take more of the drug to achieve the same effect. Jake's tolerance to cannabis means that he has been smoking more, as well as more often. He is at risk of becoming dependent on cannabis unless he finds other ways to manage his anxiety. In the long run, psychological techniques – teaching him skills to control his anxiety – will be much more helpful than psychoactive drugs.

Some people use drugs to take away very difficult, distressing feelings that they struggle with every day. The despair of depression, traumatic memories or the emotional pain of a recent bereavement, for example, are feelings that can lead people to the psychologically soothing effects of psychoactive drugs. In the short term, psychoactive drugs can make difficult feelings less intense or disappear altogether, but of course the drugs won't address the underlying problems, only mask them.

Drugs to numb physical problems

Psychoactive drugs change our psychological experiences, but they can change our physical experiences too. A number of powerful psychoactive drugs also reduce pain. Opioids such as codeine or benzodiazepines such as diazepam are medications with powerful psychoactive effects. When prescribed and carefully monitored for pain management, these drugs can be extremely helpful, but serious harm – including dependence – can result from their misuse.

Drugs for other reasons

Drug use is an attempt to experience new feelings or take away unwanted ones. For some users, this extends beyond the direct feeling caused by the drug. Drugs can make people feel good in other ways, offering an escape from responsibility, a personal reward or satisfaction in breaking the rules.

Drugs for social gain: peer groups and fitting in

Drugs can also make people feel good through social gain. In particular, for those who find it difficult to fit in with others, using drugs can give access to certain sub-cultures. Sub-cultures can offer a sense of belonging and identity that the user struggles to find elsewhere.

We've all heard the phrase 'falling in with a bad crowd'. Very often parents describe how their teenager was doing well until they met a new group of friends, who the parents felt were a bad influence. They believed, often correctly, that the new friend or friends introduced their child to drugs and that this was the root of the problem.

Most of us like to fit in. We are social animals and like to feel part of a group or community. Belonging feels good.

Using drugs is sometimes seen as a way to increase credibility with peers. Acts of recklessness can increase status within a peer group and be seen as mature or brave. If drug-taking is praised or admired by others, this makes the user feel good about themselves. With this social gain, it is likely that drug use will continue. For some, the social gains from drug use can be more important than the drug use itself (Oetting & Beauvais, 1987).

Hannah's story

Hannah is 15 years old and in trouble. She has been sent to see me by her exasperated parents because she has just been suspended from school for truancy and smoking cannabis. Hannah is preparing for her GCSE examinations, which are in a few months' time – or at least she should be preparing. In truth, she has not even started her exam revision and seems to accept that she will fail everything.

As Hannah and I begin to talk, she tells me that she feels like a 'freak' at school because her interests and musical tastes are different from those of her classmates. Hannah believes she has never really fitted in and has only recently found people like her.

These new friends come from outside her school and are slightly older than her. Most of them have already left school and are looking for work. They share Hannah's passion for electronic dance music and the culture surrounding it, and spend time listening to and making music. Hannah will often leave school after lunch to spend time with them, something she finds exciting.

I ask Hannah about drugs and she explains that she doesn't really like them, but has smoked quite a lot of cannabis with her new friends 'because that's what they do'. The cannabis makes her anxious and gives her a headache but she never refuses, as 'that would be really uncool'. Hannah's classmates know about her drug use and now avoid her even more than usual.

When I ask what she thinks will happen next, Hannah becomes very distressed and starts crying. She explains that she feels trapped, disliked at school but out of her depth with her new friends. She is worried about the cannabis and has felt quite paranoid the past few times she smoked the drug, believing that the police somehow knew what she was doing. She doesn't feel able to refuse cannabis from her new friends, as she is desperate not to be rejected by yet another group of people. Hannah is also frightened because some of the new group use 'stronger' drugs. Although she has not been offered these other drugs yet, she knows it is only a matter of time.

It becomes clear that Hannah is very unhappy both at school and at home. She is intensely lonely and very sensitive to rejection by others. Importantly, Hannah knows that her life is 'going wrong' but doesn't know what to do about it.

This was the first of many meetings I had with Hannah, meetings that also came to involve her parents, the school, a family therapist and a social worker. Hannah dropped down a school year and, at the time of writing, is still in treatment, not using drugs and making steady progress.

Some groups are particularly vulnerable to drug misuse. Children with existing emotional difficulties or problems with learning or social interaction can, without appropriate help, find environments such as school extremely challenging. This can lead them to seek out peers who also feel disenfranchised and left on the social margins. Conditions such as autism spectrum disorder and attention-deficit hyperactivity disorder (ADHD) are increasingly recognised, and children with these problems need proper assessment and support.

For those experiencing emotional distress, psychoactive drugs can seem particularly appealing. Intoxication can provide a brief refuge from difficult thoughts and feelings and so it is perhaps no surprise that children who have experienced neglect or abuse are at greater risk of drug misuse. Unfortunately, there is not enough space here to explore the social and cultural challenges of disadvantaged children or how best to meet their needs. It is an important area worthy of its own book.

Key messages

- People use psychoactive drugs to change the way they feel.
- Psychoactive drug use can result in new feelings that would otherwise be hard to experience, or take away unwanted feelings.
- Sometimes psychoactive drugs are used for social gain, bringing a sense of belonging and identity.

Drug use and adolescence

Do you remember your adolescence? Was it a period of gentle, steady maturing or a storm of intense, confusing emotions? For many people it will have been a mixture. What about your own children? Most parents notice changes as their children progress through adolescence. They might become uncharacteristically irritable, over-sleep or break previously accepted rules of behaviour. Out go cuddles, 'please' and 'thank you', replaced by complaints and criticism. This dramatic change is less surprising when we understand that adolescence is a period of massive physical and mental change.

Imagine how it feels for the adolescent. They suddenly find themselves having to cope with intense new emotions, a rapidly changing body and impulses and drives that are confusing and often contradictory. Without a guidebook or instruction manual, they manage by relying on trial and error. Just when they most need the stability and guidance of those around them, their peers are going through the same thing and their parents are missing their sweet, obedient pre-adolescent child. It is perhaps unsurprising, in this roller coaster of change, when the adolescent angrily tells their parents 'you just don't understand!'

In this chapter, we will focus on the impact of drug use during adolescence. As we will see later, the adolescent brain is especially vulnerable to the harmful effects of drugs, just at the time when drug use is most likely. But why are adolescents at such a high risk of experimenting with drugs and so susceptible to their harmful effects? Before we answer these questions, let's first try to understand what is going on in the young brain.

What is adolescence?

Some have argued that adolescence is not a specific developmental stage but instead an invention of marketing executives looking to sell their products and extract money from parents. Music, fashion, literature and food have all been aimed with increasing precision at the teen market. Most parents will recognise the plea for the latest must-have electronic device or branded clothing, without which social exclusion and humiliation are certain.

When it comes to drugs, the marketing strategies are surprisingly similar. In the legal market, alcopops (alcoholic drinks with added flavours and packaging to appeal to younger drinkers) have been heavily marketed to young people. This strategy is mimicked by 'head shops' and online sites, which market so-called 'legal highs' using brightly coloured labels and cartoons to attract younger users. The 'legal highs' can be considered the alcopops of the drug world.

But adolescence isn't just a marketing trick. Researchers describe it as a clear developmental phase (Blakemore & Choudhury, 2006). It is the bridge between childhood and adulthood, involves a complex emotional, physical and social journey, and happens in every culture.

Changes associated with adolescence

Adolescence is generally defined as the period between the onset of puberty and the point at which adult roles are assumed. For girls, this is typically between the ages of 10 and 17 years and for boys, between the ages of 12 and 18 years. It is a period of rapid transition, including physical, psychological and social changes, led by enormous development in the brain.

Physically, the body grows rapidly and organs develop. Most strikingly, the hormonal changes of puberty begin and the body starts to change from child to adult. Many parents only become aware of these changes when their previously sweet-smelling child develops pungent new odours.

Psychologically, adolescence is often caricatured as a period of irritability, moodiness and self-absorption. Professor Sarah-Jayne Blakemore illustrated this intense self-absorption during a discussion session by quoting a diary entry of an adolescent girl from 1969 (*The Psychologist*, 2015). Compared with the importance of developing relationships, world events are very much in the background:

> '20 July 1969. I went to arts center (by myself!) in yellow cords and blouse. Ian was there but he didn't speak to me. Got rhyme put in my handbag from someone who's apparently got a crush on me. It's Nicholas I think. UGH. Man landed on moon.'

Socially, adolescents begin to seek independence from their family to explore and test out their expanding physical and psychological skills. Relationships to family members may seem to fall in value, particularly when compared with new and often intense bonds with peers. Complex social networks develop, requiring new skills and understanding. Children cannot become independent of their parents without learning and practising these new skills. Adolescence is the period when these skills are fine-tuned in preparation for leaving home and exploring the world.

But the most remarkable changes of all are taking place in the adolescent brain. Changes in both the structure and function of different brain areas underpin the wider developments of adolescence. These brain changes provide clues to understanding the risks drugs pose during this period.

The plastic brain

From birth, we decide what to do on the basis of feedback. Behaviours that lead to positive outcomes are repeated, but we soon give up on behaviours that don't seem to work. Babies cry when hungry because they have learned – by repeating the behaviour – that crying is a very effective way of being noticed and getting fed.

A 6-month-old child will repeatedly push a cup off its tray table and watch with amazement and pleasure as it falls to the floor with a clatter. The child's fundamental understanding of gravity is developing. Repeating behaviours strengthens the child's understanding of cause and effect.

As the child grows, the fundamental rules of safe living are established. By testing and re-testing, patterns emerge. Very hot things burn and should be avoided, eating when hungry is satisfying and seeking cuddles and kisses feels pleasurable and reassuring.

At a brain level, these experiences are recorded and stored using groups of brain cells, known as neural networks. Large numbers of brain cells link together to form complex networks between different parts of the brain (see Chapter 4). Strongly positive experiences (e.g. eating when hungry) and negative experiences (e.g. touching hot things) are learnt by strengthening these networks. Experiences that don't lead to significant positive or negative feelings tend to have much weaker neural networks. They are less important to our understanding of the world.

Our brains keep on learning throughout our life. As we become more sociable and independent, we develop a more nuanced understanding of the world. Our repertoire of behaviours also rapidly develops in response to social interactions. This allows us to develop complex relationships with others. The brain continually learns from all these new experiences and does so by developing increasingly complex neural networks.

These networks can be modified by new experiences allowing new behaviours to take the place of old ones. This has led researchers to describe our brains as flexible and as having 'plasticity'. Rather than learning being fixed once and for all, our brain continually adds new information by constantly updating and modifying the neural networks. Plasticity allows us to learn from our mistakes. Adolescence is a critical period for developing and fine-tuning new, healthy, successful behaviours and the brain is ready to record successes and learn from mistakes.

How the brain grows during adolescence

The brain grows throughout childhood and the number of neurons (brain cells) slowly increases. With the beginning of puberty, however, this number peaks. There is no other period in our lives when we will have as many brain cells! The process then goes into reverse and the brain actually begins to lose cells, a process researchers describe as synaptic pruning.

How is it that, during a period when the adolescent brain is building and strengthening the neural networks, the number of neurons is decreasing? The most likely answer is that the brain is beginning to sort out what is and isn't important by 'culling' cells that it doesn't need. It might be losing brain cells, but it is strengthening the most important neural networks.

The brain develops in a specific order. The complex networks linking different parts of the brain need to grow not only at the right pace but also in the correct order.

Impulsivity and the adolescent brain

Curiously, the brain develops from back to front. One of the last areas in the adolescent brain to mature are the frontal lobes, which are responsible for conscious decision-making (Blakemore & Choudhury, 2006). This is the area that carefully weighs up the benefits and risks of an action. The frontal lobes put the brakes on impulsive or dangerous decisions. However, while the frontal lobes are still developing, other parts of the brain are racing ahead. One such area is the striatum, which is the novelty-seeking and reward centre of the brain. A balance between frontal lobes and striatum is thought to be crucial for self-control.

In an adult brain, the frontal lobes are ready to moderate impulsive behaviours. Activities that might seem attractive and exciting in the moment will often be avoided if they have significant risk attached. For the adolescent brain, however, the striatum is unopposed by the still-developing frontal lobes. There are no mental brakes to protect against rash decisions.

Could the impulsive adolescent brain be an advantage?

It would be easy to see the adolescent brain, with its apparent poor self-control, as leading the adolescent into risk and danger, but could there be any advantages to being more impulsive? Do our brains develop this way for a reason?

Some researchers think so, suggesting that impulsivity and novelty-seeking has a purpose (Steinberg, 2008; Crone & Dahl, 2012). Adolescents need to experience new things and take some risks to learn about the world. Without getting things wrong and making mistakes, adolescents won't be able to test out their new skills and develop judgement. Just like a small child has to find out that hot things burn and ceramic cups break when dropped on tiled floors, an adolescent must also learn about more complicated issues through trial and error.

This puts parents in a difficult situation. On the one hand, we try to provide an environment that is safe and secure, while on the other we need to let our children take enough risks to learn and develop. To make the task even harder, the balance of risk and safety needs to be constantly adjusted. The right balance for a 14-year-old will be wrong for a 16-year-old.

Why using drugs in adolescence is a really bad idea

As we have seen, the adolescent brain develops in a way that makes risk-taking and novelty-seeking more likely. Lacking the brain maturity and experience to support good judgement, there is no time when drug use is more likely. But during this critical period of development, the adolescent brain seems to be most vulnerable to the harmful effects of drugs. Drugs can damage the structure and functioning of the brain, disrupting the developing neural networks (Realini *et al*, 2009).

Worse still, heavy drug use may lead to brain changes that increase the likelihood of further drug use. This is double trouble for the adolescent brain. Poor decision-making leads to drug use, then the drugs themselves damage the brain, leading to further drug use.

Key messages

- Adolescence is the period between the onset of puberty and the point at which adult roles are assumed and involves rapid physical, psychological and social change.

- In adolescence, learning takes place as the brain establishes neural networks. These networks are constantly modified by new experiences.

- The adolescent brain develops in stages. One of the last areas to develop are the frontal lobes, the part of the brain responsible for decision-making and assessing risk.

- Just when the adolescent brain is at this delicate developmental phase, it is also most impulsive and drug use is most likely.

- Drug use in adolescence disrupts brain development, which can lead to long-term damage to brain function and increase the risk of further drug use.

How much do adolescents know about their drugs?

Psychoactive substances are widely available, whether from friends, dealers or online. If your child decides to experiment with drugs, finding some won't be difficult.

Most children don't ever try drugs, but a significant minority do. As we have established, around one in five people in the UK who are 16–24 years of age used a drug in the past year (Home Office, 2014). I am often surprised by how little the young people I see in my practice know about the drugs they are taking or the risks.

William's story

William is a 15-year-old schoolboy. He has asked his parents if he can 'see someone about my head' but insisted he come to the appointment alone.

He arrives early and looks worried. William speaks clearly and thoughtfully about his problems, explaining that for 3 months he has experienced paranoia. He believes his friends may be plotting against him and that they steal things from his room at night when he is asleep. In the classroom, he overhears snatches of conversation making fun of him. Last week he noticed people in the street staring at him and wondered if they had talked to his school friends and were 'in on it'.

William finds these thoughts very distressing. Sometimes he is convinced the thoughts are true, while at other times he thinks his mind is 'playing tricks' and it is all in his head. William is worried he is 'going mad'.

I ask William about drugs and he explains that he has been smoking synthetic cannabis, which he buys from the internet. He says the synthetic cannabis 'relaxes my brain' and takes away the distressing thoughts. William has been smoking synthetic cannabis for about 6 months. The persecutory thoughts developed after he started taking the drug.

When I ask William to tell me more about his cannabis use, he seems surprised I'm so interested. He says he initially found synthetic cannabis enjoyable and relaxing but felt it was much stronger than the natural cannabis he used to smoke.

After a month of using synthetic cannabis 'most days', he began to experience persecutory thinking. William found that immediately after smoking synthetic cannabis, the persecutory thinking improved and he felt more relaxed for a few hours. 'I feel better when I'm a bit stoned. It gives me a break from it all', he says.

I ask William what he knows about synthetic cannabis and if he thinks it might be contributing to his persecutory symptoms. His answer is interesting. First, he says that synthetic cannabis is legal and because of this he believes it is unlikely to cause any serious harm. 'They would ban it if it made you go crazy,' he reasons. Second, because it was synthetic, rather than natural, he thinks of it as 'pure' and less likely to cause problems. Third, a close friend had told him it would help him relax and make him feel better, which was very much William's experience. Synthetic cannabis seems to be a good relaxant and, better still, it makes the persecutory thoughts go away for a few hours.

William and I talk about possible reasons for the persecutory thinking. A wide range of issues can cause the problems he describes, from intense anxiety and stress to severe mental illness such as schizophrenia.

Synthetic cannabis can also lead to persecutory thinking, possibly more often than natural cannabis. William felt better immediately after smoking synthetic cannabis so had slowly increased the amount he used. Unfortunately, his persecutory thinking had also slowly increased.

When asked about his family history, William tells me that an uncle of his had 'gone mad' and spent time receiving treatment in a psychiatric hospital. He doesn't know any more detail.

I suggest that the synthetic cannabis could be the cause of his symptoms and we talk about how we could know for sure. William agrees that the only way to find out is to stop using it and see what happens. He agrees to stop all synthetic cannabis for 3 weeks and to keep a diary rating how bad the persecutory symptoms are each day. William expects the persecutory thinking to get worse without the help of the synthetic cannabis, but is willing to try.

William returns to see me a few weeks later. To his surprise, his symptoms improved greatly when he stopped using cannabis. He is delighted and now wants to stop using the drug for good. He is also hugely relieved. He had looked at his symptoms on the internet and, although he hadn't admitted it when we first met, was terrified that he had developed schizophrenia. We agree that the synthetic cannabis was the most likely cause of his symptoms.

William may carry a genetic vulnerability to experiencing paranoia when he takes drugs and his uncle's illness should be treated as a warning sign. William says he is going to avoid drugs 'at all costs'.

A few weeks later, William calls to let me know that he has not used any more cannabis. The persecutory thinking has completely disappeared and he feels 'back to normal'.

William's story shows how poor knowledge about drugs can lead to further harm. For William, his lack of knowledge led him to increase his drug use to treat symptoms the drug was actually causing in the first place. A lack of knowledge is dangerous, but misinformation is just as harmful.

A recent example is the dissociative drug, methoxetamine, known to many users as 'mexxy'. Methoxetamine appeared on the drug scene at a time when users were becoming aware that a more popular drug, ketamine, could cause severe bladder damage. Methoxetamine was marketed by the dealers as cheaper than ketamine, just as powerful, but with none of the harmful bladder effects. Several of my patients switched to this new drug, convinced that it was safer. Without any other information, they chose to trust the dealer's sales pitch. As methoxetamine became more popular, it became clear that it damaged the bladder in a similar way to ketamine (Dargan *et al*, 2014), as well as having other severe, unwanted effects. Methoxetamine use has now plummeted in the UK.

What's interesting about the methoxetamine example is that users accepted information from drug dealers at face value. The dealers said what the users wanted to hear, and very few users looked for information to back up the dealers' claims. This is a real challenge for clinicians, because information influences behaviour. Users need accurate, credible information to make informed choices. The information battle lines are drawn between the dealer's pitch and health research, with hearsay and rumour often ruling the day.

The mystery white powder

But what if users don't care what drug they are taking? Over the past few years, there has been an increase in people using what some researchers call 'mystery white powder' with generic names such as 'bubble'. Probably a blend of synthetic stimulant drugs (Measham *et al*, 2011), mystery white powder finds a market in people who don't seem to care what drug they are consuming, as long as it is cheap and effective.

Where do drug users get their information?

These examples raise interesting questions about where drug users get information about drugs. Table 2.1 shows the results of European research exploring this question (European Commission, 2014). Over 13 000 15- to 24-year-olds in the European Union were asked where they would go for information about illicit drugs. Respondents could choose more than one answer. The internet, including chat rooms, came top, with 60% choosing this option. A third of people said they would ask their friends, and a quarter would talk to their parents or relatives.

Meeting the information challenge: harnessing the internet

Getting accurate information about drugs to those who use them is a problem. Accurate information challenges the many drug myths and helps users make better choices. Even if someone decides to keep using drugs, there is usually helpful information available about using them more safely. But reaching drug users with accurate information is difficult. As the methoxetamine example illustrated, people tend to believe what they want to believe.

Table 2.1 Where people 15–24 years of age get information about drugs

Source	Proportion of respondents
Internet	59%
A friend	36%
Health professional	31%
Parent or relative	25%
Specialist drug counsellor or centre	21%
Police	13%
Media	10%
Someone at school or work	9%
Youth or social worker	7%
Telephone helpline	4%

Source: European Commission (2014).

There are numerous chat rooms and online forums dedicated to drugs and drug use. Health services have yet to take full advantage of the internet as a tool to reach users, but this may be the clinician's best chance to usefully promote accurate information about drugs. See the Appendix for a list of reputable online resources for parents and adolescents.

Key messages

- Many adolescents are surprisingly poorly informed about drugs, their effects and the harms they can cause.
- Adolescents tend to seek information about drugs from the internet or friends.
- Accurate information is available, but adolescents often don't know where to find it.

Having the drug conversation with your child

Good information is critical in decision-making. If you don't have the right information, how can you weigh up the risks and benefits of different choices? The challenge for parents is not just to provide the correct information, but to do so in a way that your child will pay attention to it.

For some parents, talking to their child about drugs is relatively easy, but for others it's awkward and embarrassing. It is a good idea to start talking to children about drugs before they come into contact with them or people who are using them. Having the right information early on will help them weigh up the risks and might stop them from even trying drugs. If they do choose to use drugs, good-quality information may help them reduce the risk.

Just as importantly, by talking with your child about drugs, you help them understand that this is a topic you know something about and you're happy to talk about, and that you might even be a source of good advice if problems arise.

Do I really need to talk to my child about drugs? Won't the school do it?

Many schools provide information to children about drugs, either from people within the school or by bringing in outside speakers. However, there are no specific requirements for UK schools to deliver a particular programme. Instead schools are given the flexibility to tailor their local personal, social, health and economic (PSHE) education programmes to reflect the needs of their students. Government guidance states that schools should 'use their PSHE education programme to equip pupils with a sound understanding of risk and with the knowledge and skills necessary to make safe and informed decisions' (Department for Education, 2013). Although the PSHE curriculum suggests covering the topic of drugs, schools do not have to. Drug education is a required part of the science curriculum, which begins in Year 6 (when students are 10 or 11 years of age).

Unfortunately, it is not clear which is the best way to teach children about drugs. Research suggests that teaching all children about drugs may not be the most effective approach (Faggiano *et al*, 2014). The majority of children don't try drugs. They have already made a decision that it is not for them and education is unlikely to have any impact on their behaviour. Instead of offering drug education to all children, some experts have suggested targeting vulnerable children to improve their resilience and decision-making (National Institute for Health and Care Excellence, 2007*a*).

It's also unclear what content drug education should include. Some suggest that the best approach is to frighten children with horror stories of the harmful effects of drugs, but experts believe that this approach is at best ineffective and at worse actually increases drug use (Advisory Council on the Misuse of Drugs, 2015). In the UK, Mentor-ADEPIS has developed quality standards for drug education that are based on the best evidence currently available (Mentor-ADEPIS, 2014).

What is important is that the information your child hears is accurate and consistent. It will confuse them if what they are being told at school is different to what they are hearing at home. Check with your child's school to see what is being taught about drugs.

For some parents, it may seem reasonable to leave drug education to their child's school, particularly if they feel the school is doing a good job and they don't know much about drugs themselves. But there are good reasons why parents should have the drug conversation with their child.

Why you should talk to your child about drugs before they are exposed to them

Parents matter

As a parent, you are an incredibly important and influential figure in your child's life. Your job is to support and guide them as they make the transition from childhood to adulthood. They have grown up under your care and during that time have taken on and accepted many of your values and beliefs. Children learn from their own experiences but also by observing others, a process known as vicarious learning. They have spent more time with you than anyone and as a result have learnt more from you than from anyone else. Your views on what is acceptable and how you respond to positive and negative experiences will have been closely observed by them throughout their childhood and much of what you do will be copied (or modelled) by your child as they grow up. Younger children assume that their parents are always right and believe most of what they say. Without knowing much about the outside world, they let their parents fill in the gaps for them.

But during adolescence, when your child is becoming more independent, there is a natural and normal process of testing out and challenging parental values and beliefs. The adolescent begins to make their own judgements about the world around them. This is often experienced by parents as rejection or even hostility, particularly when children start questioning accepted truths and family values. For children, this process of challenging and breaking the rules is a critical part of development. You may feel your views have lost their influence, and in part this is true, but that undervalues all your years of nurturing. Whether your adolescent agrees with you or not, what you say still matters.

Andy and Jane's story

Andy and Jane have made an appointment to see me abou their 14-year-old daugher, Abby, but arrive on their own. They are worried about Abby. Over the past 6 months, Abby has become increasingly withdrawn at home and at school. The school is also concerned because Abby's academic performance has slumped. Andy and Jane first thought it was all to do with her boyfriend, John. Although they liked John, they worried that he was 'a bit wild'. The relationship broke up a few weeks ago and Abby seemed surprisingly unaffected.

Andy and Jane have clear views about drugs and think that any use is unacceptable and dangerous. Neither of them have ever used illegal drugs of any sort. They were shocked when last week they found cannabis in Abby's bedroom, but when they confronted her, she said it was not hers but that she was 'holding it' for a friend. She promised them that she had not touched it, but refused to take a drug test that Andy bought online. Abby also refused to come to today's appointment, saying that it was 'a waste of time'.

Both parents feel they have lost their connection with Abby and don't know how to re-engage with her. They feel frightened and out of their depth regarding the cannabis and don't know what to do next. They have never spoken to Abby about drugs before and don't know how to begin a conversation now. All they really want to say to her is that taking drugs is 'stupid and dangerous' and that they are angry and disappointed.

As the session continues, I learn that both parents have a rather distant relationship to Abby. Although they clearly love her very much, they have tended to let her get on with things and have never had a close physical relationship. Cuddles ended early and both Andy and Jane find talking about 'emotional things' awkward and embarrassing. They both grew up in families where discussing feelings was frowned upon and seen as something of a weakness. Andy and Jane parented Abby as they had been parented themselves and felt comfortable with this. When Abby began to challenge family rules, it became clear they didn't really understand her emotional world very well, but didn't know how to do things differently. They both feel stuck and frightened.

Towards the end of the session, we discuss how I might help. They do not think Abby will come to an appointment, so instead we talk about how I can support them in helping her. The challenge for Andy and Jane is to talk to Abby so they can understand what is going on and help Abby through what sounds like a difficult period. We carefully plan a series of conversations for them to have with their daughter.

At home, Andy and Jane are surprised to find Abby is receptive to talking with them and quickly discover that Abby has been unhappy for a long time. She admits using cannabis, saying that it takes away 'horrible thoughts' she has about her weight. Abby also discloses that she has been superficially cutting her arms and that this has both frightened and excited her. Abby is relieved to be able to share her feelings and asks if Andy and Jane can speak to the school about her problems, which they do.

When Andy and Jane first came to see me, they were overwhelmed with emotions and didn't know how to help their daughter. With only very simple guidance, including some role-play, they began talking with Abby. Through these conversations they realised that Abby was feeling isolated and lonely and was desperate to ask them for advice.

With support from the school counsellor and her parents, Abby decided to stop using cannabis. She was referred to a clinical psychologist to talk about her perceived weight problem and better ways to control her feelings than self-harm. She is still in treatment and making good progress.

Many parents, like Andy and Jane, feel ill-equipped to help their child. They feel that they no longer have any influence and don't know what to do. If you feel this way, I encourage you to pause, take stock and remember that what you say still matters, even when communication between you and your child is less than perfect.

The first step is to put your emotions to one side and listen carefully to what your child is saying. You will probably feel that your child is not listening to you, and in the middle of a heated argument you might be right! However, consistent, clear messages have a way of sinking in, especially if they are coming from someone who has been a reliable presence throughout the child's life.

It's good to talk

By raising the subject yourself, you are letting your child know that talking about drugs is acceptable. It is much more difficult to engage your child in a conversation about drugs if the first time you raise the issue is in the middle of a crisis. It is far better for the subject to have already been put on the table, so you can get on with helping them, rather than awkwardly trying to figure out what to say.

Developing a genuine dialogue with your child about drugs can be very challenging and there will be anxiety for both parties about feeling unheard, patronised or punished. However, if problems do develop, as a parent you will be on the front line. Others may be there to support and help you, but most parents feel that they are responsible for sorting things out. Communication then becomes critical and, although the conversations may be very difficult, the more open the communication the more a parent can help their child.

Information influences choice

The decision to use drugs depends on many things, including price, perceived benefit, context, peer pressure, previous experience and potential risk. Having accurate information about the effects and risks of using drugs is important, because this information will be part of making a decision to use or not. For adolescents who are already using drugs, it might help them use more safely, reduce their use, or stop altogether. Accurate information will help your child make better decisions.

You may be confident that you already have sufficient knowledge about drugs, but if not it is worth knowing the best place to find it. Remember there is a huge amount of misinformation available about drugs, particularly on the internet, and that this could be where your child educates themself. Consider directing your child to reliable sources of information, even if they choose to compare this information with other, less accurate sources. See Chapter 4 for a description of how drugs work in the brain, Chapter 5 for a summary of the different types of drugs and the Appendix for a list of reliable online sources.

How to start the drug conversation

When starting the drug conversation, a common worry for parents is that they don't know enough about drugs. They fear that their adolescent will wince with embarrassment, mock their lack of knowledge and refuse to listen to them. Many parents will never have tried a psychoactive drug themselves (excluding alcohol, caffeine and tobacco) and so feel they don't have enough experience to have a meaningful discussion.

On the other hand, some parents will have experimented with drugs at some point in their life and may feel able to speak with great authority. A word of caution for these parents – drug culture changes quickly and both the drugs and the way they are used may now be different.

Many of my adolescent patients talk with amusement about the time their parents first spoke to them about drugs. However, they also usually appreciated that their parents were prepared to have the conversation and were often surprised by how well-informed they were. Unless told otherwise, children generally assume their parents have never even seen a drug, let alone used one.

It's a conversation, not a lecture

The drug conversation should not be a lecture. It is a two-way discussion with the aim of helping your child make good choices and reduce their risk of harm. You want to show your child that this is an important topic you are willing and able to talk about.

Explain your own views on drugs, whatever they might be, ideally in a way that allows for further discussion. Different parents will have different views on drugs, some of it gained from personal experience. Many parents will oppose drug use of any sort. Others may feel that experimentation with 'soft' drugs such as cannabis is acceptable but that 'harder' drugs are to be avoided at all costs.

Whatever your opinion, how you have the conversation is crucial. Saying that you completely disapprove of all drug use is fine, but consider adding some context. You may have had personal experience with a family member or friend having drug-related problems and this will help your child understand where your opinion comes from. It is particularly important to let your child know if there is any family history of drug or alcohol problems, as they may be carrying a genetic vulnerability to drug problems. If your child is weighing up the risk of using drugs, this is crucial information.

You might say you are against drug use because it can be dangerous. If this is your opinion, have some information at hand regarding the risks. Be careful not to exaggerate risks or say anything that is untrue. Telling your child that ecstasy is very likely to kill them could backfire if your child sees friends using the drug without any obvious harm. It is far better to provide them with a realistic and credible summary of the risks.

It is also important to ask your child questions and listen to what they have to say. Do they know anyone who uses drugs? How do they feel about that? You may not have much idea what sort of drugs people are currently using, especially with the number of new drugs constantly increasing. Instead of guessing, try asking your child what drugs they have heard about. Is drug use seen as exciting, glamorous and grown up or dangerous and harmful? Have they ever been offered drugs? If so, did they feel any pressure to accept? Depending on their age and openness, these questions and others may help you understand the drug 'landscape' your child inhabits.

When is the best time to begin the drug conversation?

A conversation about drugs will be more difficult if a child is already using them and experiencing problems. By then, family relationships are often under severe strain, opinions about what should be done become increasingly polarised and the emotional intensity can become overwhelming. This would not be the ideal situation in which to have a calm, reasoned conversation about drugs.

It is best to talk to your child about drugs earlier, rather than later. There is no clear evidence on the best time to do this, but from my experience, it would be around the time that they first become aware of drugs. They might hear about drugs from the media or in the playground. It is important to talk to your children before they are actually exposed to drugs or to people who are using drugs.

The timing of the conversation will also depend on the maturity of your child, whether they have older siblings and how common drug use is in your community. Children mature at different rates, but most children will receive some education about drugs from around the 11 years of age and may be talking about drugs with their friends well before that. Around 10 or 11 years of age is a reasonable time to have a first conversation for most children.

If you are aware of particular risks, such as a strong family history of drug or alcohol problems, or feel that your child is at greater risk than other children, then you might decide to begin a discussion earlier. It is better to have this conversation before they are exposed to drugs or people who use drugs.

The dos and don'ts of having the drug conversation

A conversation between a parent and adolescent about drug use is rather like the conversation about safe sex. It has the potential for excruciating embarrassment on both sides and because of this tends to be avoided. But, however tricky, it is an important conversation to have, even if it is only once and then joked about for years afterwards. So, what should you say?

Don't feel it all has to be said in one conversation

The first conversation may be the only one, or it may lead to further conversations. Once the topic has been put on the table, it is much easier to talk about it as need arises.

Do set the scene

Find the right moment. This is an important conversation and you don't want to be interrupted. Alert your child that you want to talk to them about something important, but that they're not in trouble. You might want to give them advance notice, explaining that later that day you want to sit down with them to talk about drugs.

Do think about whether one parent or both should be involved

Depending on your child's age and the nature of your relationship with the other parent, if there is one around, you have to decide whether one or both of you will be involved in the conversation. Talking with both parents might be too intimidating for some children. If only one parent has the conversation, it is important that your child knows that both parents have agreed and that the other parent is aware that this conversation is taking place. This is particularly important if parents are not living together. Depending on the structure of the family, sometimes other family members or even family friends might be better placed than a parent to have the conversation.

Do be clear what the conversation is about

From the beginning, be clear what you want to talk about and why it is important. It's also important to stick to the topic. You might start the conversation with the best of intentions but, because it is an unfamiliar, awkward topic, quickly move on to discuss something else. One way to avoid this is to be clear what points you want to cover before you start. Although you want to have a two-way conversation, rather than a lecture, sometimes it is helpful to have a checklist of points written down to make sure you don't forget anything.

Do be consistent

Consistent messages are key. It can be very confusing for a child if their parents have different opinions on topics such as drugs and parents can sometimes give different messages without meaning to. It is best for parents to agree on the messages before they speak to their child.

Do keep calm and listen

It is not normal to talk about drugs and it can be very easy for the conversation to become emotional and the viewpoints of parent and child polarised. Approach the conversation in a calm manner. Your intention should be to have a discussion that helps your child make better choices and opens communication with them on an issue they will inevitably come across at some point. What you say is important, but what they say is even more so. Make sure they have a chance to comment on what you have said and listen carefully to what they say.

Don't accuse

Your child might be surprised, embarrassed or assume you are talking to them because you think they are using drugs. If you start young enough, this is less likely. It might be good to start the conversation by saying that they will come across drugs at some point and that is why it is important that they know something about them. If you think your child has already tried drugs, you might need to approach the conversation differently.

In this situation, it is especially important to avoid accusations if the conversation it to be successful. Chapter 7 will focus on what to do if you think your child is using drugs.

Don't interrogate

It's easy for a parent to start a well-intentioned conversation but for it to rapidly turn into an interrogation. Try hard to avoid this. No one likes to be put on the spot and it will reduce, rather than increase, the chance of further honest dialogue. If your child is open to talking about drugs, then start with less personal questions. For example, ask if they know anyone who has used drugs, perhaps in the year above or outside of school. Other good opening questions include asking them how much they know about drugs, what they've been taught in school and where would they look for information if they wanted to know more. Your child may already have strong opinions on drugs, so consider asking them what they think about people who use them.

Don't claim ignorance or pretend to know everything

If you say you don't know anything about drugs, your child could reasonably question on what authority you are now speaking to them. But don't pretend to know everything, either. Whatever your own previous experience of drugs, you are having this conversation as a parent, not as an expert on drugs. Your child might be suspicious or feel alarmed if you show an encyclopaedic knowledge of drugs and their effects. Depending on the age of your child, they may be shocked you even know what drugs are. It is important to say that you don't know everything but that you do know where to get reliable information.

Do give them information

One of the most helpful things you can do is point your child in the direction of good information. The drug market can change quickly and new drugs are emerging all the time. Having an easily accessible source of up-to-date information can be very helpful for your child. Some good sources are listed in the Appendix.

Don't forget alcohol

By far the most commonly used psychoactive drug is alcohol. Although this book does not cover alcohol in detail, like other psychoactive drugs, alcohol can be harmful both in the short term and with longer-term use. It's used for the same reasons as other drugs – to give new feelings or to take away feelings that aren't wanted. Many parents will feel much more comfortable talking about alcohol than drugs because it is legal and they have greater knowledge and experience. Alcohol mixes dangerously with most psychoactive drugs and this is important information your child should know.

Do make sure you leave plenty of time for questions

Talking to your child about drugs and directing them to accurate information is important. The conversation is also a chance for your child to ask you questions. They may have heard stories about drugs from their peers, school and the media. Give your child the chance to ask questions about what they've heard as well as any other questions they may have. If you don't know the answer, don't bluff. Say you don't know the answer but will find out and let them know.

Do be prepared for tricky questions

You are unlikely to have the drug conversation without being asked if you have ever used drugs yourself. Decide what you are going to say about your experience with drugs before you start the conversation. If you have used drugs in the past, then you need to decide whether to disclose this or not. For younger children, it may be confusing for them to hear you say that drugs are harmful and then admit to using them yourself. For adolescents, the same may apply, but in some cases a more open conversation can help de-stigmatise the issue. Consider what you are going to say carefully before you speak to your child, as children are alarmingly good at spotting evasion.

Do leave the door open for further talks

Whether your conversation has gone well or not, end by offering a further time to discuss this topic. Your child might need time to absorb what's been said. It is good to have a follow-up conversation within a week or so, to see if your child has any more questions or wants to talk about anything further. Make it clear that you are happy to talk again at any point in the future. If the other parent is not present, then explain that they are happy to do this as well (assuming this is possible and is the case).

Do finish with praise

However well (or badly) the conversation with your child went, explain that you are pleased that you have been able to talk with them. For younger children in particular, however much they engaged, praise them for being able to have such a grown-up conversation. They will have found it hard work too!

Getting it wrong

Helen and Mike's story

Helen and Mike have two children: Ella, who is 14 years old and Harry, who is 10 years old. Helen is a solicitor and Mike runs his own business. Neither of them has ever used drugs.

Over the past 6 months, the couple has been increasingly worried about Ella. She has become withdrawn, spending most of her time in her bedroom. Two weekends ago, Ella came home from an afternoon with friends smelling of alcohol. When Helen challenged her, she became angry, went to her room and slammed her door. The next morning, she apologised, saying that someone had spiked her soft drink with vodka.

Mike reassured Helen that it was common for teenagers to try alcohol and remembered doing the same himself at that age without any problems. He felt Ella's behaviour was just part of normal experimentation. Helen disagreed, and was worried that Ella was now withdrawn and hard to talk to. She thought Ella might be using drugs, as another parent at the school had a similar experience with her daughter, who was using cannabis. The couple agreed that it was important to work out how often Ella was drinking and if she was using drugs.

That evening, Helen knocks on Ella's door. Ella is online chatting to friends and looks startled by her mother appearing in her bedroom.

Helen: Hi Ella, listen, I really need to talk to you about something important. Can you switch off your laptop for a second so we can talk?

Ella: What is it? Am I in trouble?

Helen: I want to talk to you about drugs. They're everywhere and I want to make sure you know about them. So you know how dangerous they are.

Ella: (Rolls her eyes and groans) I don't use drugs, Mum. Is that it?

Helen: Well, yes, OK. I just wanted to check, I am your mother. If you ever think of using them, please speak to me before you do, they are dangerous and you never know what you are really taking.

Ella: I'm not using drugs. Have you finished? I've got homework to do.

Helen: Yes, OK. I just thought it was important to ask. Now, what would you like for dinner?

The conversation ends there and Helen later admits to Mike that she didn't think it had been very helpful.

These conversations are difficult and don't always go to plan. Let's look back over the conversation between Helen and Ella. What went well and what didn't go to plan?

When Helen spoke to Ella, she sprang the conversation on her without warning. Ella assumed that she was being accused of using drugs and immediately became defensive. Before things even got going, Ella seemed to have made up her mind that she was not going to take part and the conversation fizzled out after a few brief sentences, instead moving on to the much safer topic of dinner. Helen understandably felt frustrated and that she had not achieved her aim.

What could Helen and Mike have done differently?

The couple decided to talk to Ella about alcohol and drugs, but didn't plan what they wanted to say. Being clear about their goals would have helped structure the conversation. They could, for example, have had three goals: first, asking Ella about her use of alcohol; second, understanding how much Ella knows about drugs; and third, finding out if she knows where to find accurate information. That might have been enough for the initial conversation.

It would also have been better if Helen had alerted Ella beforehand that she was going to speak to her about drugs to give her an opportunity to prepare. If Ella had not felt ambushed, she might have participated in the conversation.

On the positive side, Helen has now spoken to Ella about drugs and there is the opportunity to revisit the topic with a better-planned conversation in the future. It may be that Mike is more involved next time, either having the conversation himself or with Helen as a couple.

Getting it right

Angela's story

Angela is an estate agent who lives with her two children. Isaac is 11 years old and Julia is 9 years old. Angela was divorced 3 years ago and the children see their father, James, every other weekend. Angela and James remain on reasonable terms and speak most weeks about the children. Angela worries greatly about the impact of the divorce on her children, although both children seem to be happy, are doing well at school and have plenty of friends.

Drugs have played a huge role in Angela's life because her own brother, Jonathan, had drug problems from his teens to his mid-twenties. During that time, Jonathan's life was very chaotic. His drug use caused enormous worry and distress for his family, and Angela vividly remembers two occasions when Jonathan accidentally overdosed and she thought he would die. At 26, Jonathan began a treatment programme and stopped using drugs for good. After his treatment, he told Angela that 'drugs run in our family' and that they had an uncle who was an 'addict'. At the time, Angela promised herself that she would speak to her children about drugs and let them know about the family history.

After discussing it with James, Angela decides it's the right time to speak to her son about drugs. The following day, before Isaac goes to school, she explains that she wants to catch up with him that evening. Angela tells him he hasn't done anything wrong but that there are a few things she wanted to discuss. Isaac looks suspicious, but agrees.

That evening, after Julia had gone to bed, Angela sat down with Isaac to watch the television. The conversation went something like this:

Angela: Isaac, you know I said there were a few things I wanted to chat to you about? Do you mind if we turn off the TV for a moment and talk now? It is nothing to worry about and it won't take too long.

Isaac: (Rolls his eyes. Switches off the TV.) Mum, this is my favourite. I'm going to miss it!

Angela: This won't take long. Well, I know this is a funny thing to talk about, but I want to talk about drugs. Not medicines, but the type people take for fun.

Isaac: Mum, I know what drugs are, they told us about them in school. It was so boring, Eddie actually fell asleep in the lesson.

Angela: What did they talk to you about?

Isaac: About how they make you go mad and mess up your brain. They showed us this weird video, I can't remember that much about it. Why are you asking me?

Angela: Well, drugs are important to talk about. You will meet people who use drugs at some point and you may be offered them. I just want you to know enough about them.

Isaac: Mum, I'm not going to take drugs. Why would I?

Angela: Sometimes, if people around you are experimenting with things, it is tempting to try them as well. To be part of the crowd and fit in. Do you know anyone who uses drugs at school?

Isaac: No-one uses in my year, but some of the boys in the year above say they smoke drugs at parties. I don't really know who and I'm not sure if I believe them. Why are you so interested in drugs, Mum?

Angela: There is so much wrong information about drugs, I want to make sure you know where to read something truthful. It's always worth checking what your friends say, to make sure they really know what they are talking about. Where would you find out information about drugs if you wanted to?

Isaac: Don't know. Probably ask Eddie. He seems to know about everything.

Angela: Remember last year when Eddie told you that car sun-roofs were solar panels and you couldn't convince him they weren't? Suppose he told you something about drugs, how would you know he hadn't got it wrong?

Isaac: Yeah, I suppose.

Angela: Another reason I want to talk to you about drugs is because of Uncle Jonathan. You remember I told you he was very ill for a while?

Isaac: Yeah, he was sick and went to a hospital. Was that because of drugs?

Angela: Yes, he had a real problem with drugs. They affected him really badly and made him very sick until he got help. It is really important to know, because sometimes if one person from a family has problems with drugs, other people in the family can be more at risk as well.

Isaac: What do you mean?

Angela: Well, it means that you and Julia, and me, we may all react really badly if we ever took drugs. They might cause us bigger problems than for other people. Like a bad reaction.

Isaac: Have you ever tried drugs, Mum? Even once?

Angela: No. Seeing Uncle Jonathan getting sick convinced me never to even try them.

Isaac: OK, fine. Is Uncle Jonathan OK now?

Angela: Yes, he's fine but he still has treatment for drugs, even now all these years later. I wonder if I could give you some websites that have good information about drugs? You don't need to look at them unless you want to, but at least you have them if you need them.

Isaac: OK, Mum. Can I watch TV now?

Angela: Yes, I've been really looking forward to this series. Thanks for talking with me about this. It was really important. If you ever want to talk about it again, I'd be really happy to. Now, where's the remote control?

Angela feels relieved to have spoken with Isaac, particularly about her own brother's problems. By preparing Isaac, he didn't feel accused or caught out. He listened to what she had to say, asked questions and was able to share with her some of what he knew. Afterwards she felt much more confident about returning to the conversation in the future if needed.

What could Angela have done differently?

Angela had planned to tell Isaac that she had spoken to his father and that he knew what they were talking about, but she forgot. It would also have been good to mention alcohol as well, although that might have been too much for Isaac this time. Overall, though, Angela did very well, and should return to the subject in a week to check if Isaac has thought of any questions.

The drug conversation

1. Decide when is the right age to have the drug conversation.
2. Prepare what you are going to say, ideally with the other parent.
3. Set aside time and alert your child.
4. Be calm and consistent.
5. Begin with less personal questions, such as 'What have you learnt at school about drugs?'
6. Tell your child where they can find accurate information.
7. Mention any history of drug problems in the family.
8. Discuss alcohol.
9. Take time for questions.
10. Give praise and return to the topic in a week.

You know your child better than anyone and, although these suggestions are a helpful guide, you should think carefully about what approach your child might respond to best.

Key messages

- Talking to your child about psychoactive drugs is crucial, preferably before they are exposed to drugs or people who use them.
- As a parent, what you say matters.
- Check with the school to see what your child is being taught about drugs.
- Having the drug conversation can be difficult, but using the checklist provided will make it easier and more successful.

Drugs and the brain

To understand why people use psychoactive drugs, we need to understand how they cause their powerful effects. We will now turn our attention to how drugs work in the brain.

Drugs can change a person's mood (e.g. causing euphoria), cognition (ability to think logically), level of consciousness (from very alert to very drowsy) and behaviour (act out of character). These effects are usually the reason people take the drug in the first place. The experience of 'getting high', 'getting stoned' or 'tripping' is caused by changes in the chemical systems of the brain.

Psychoactive drugs can act in several ways.

- Stimulants make you feel excited and alert.
- Sedatives make you feel calm and relaxed.
- Hallucinogens distort how you see, hear and feel things.
- Dissociatives change your sense of yourself and your body.

Before we look at these effects, let's talk about how the brain works without drugs.

A quick tour of the brain

The brain is our most complex organ and is the body's command centre. It is divided into different sections, or lobes, which focus on particular activities.

The occipital lobes, at the rear of the brain, are involved with vision. Parts of the temporal lobes, which are at the sides of the brain, process sound, and the parietal lobes, at the top of the brain, are largely responsible for integrating sensory information relating to taste and touch. Perhaps the most important are the frontal lobes, which, as the name suggests, are located at the front of the brain directly above our eyeballs. The frontal lobes are responsible for, among other things, decision-making. This is where we balance the pros and cons of a particular action and decide if it is a good idea or not.

None of the lobes work alone. Instead, they are joined by a complex network of nerves that reaches across the brain. This network helps the brain communicate information at high speed, making it very efficient.

How the brain 'thinks'

The building blocks of this network are nerve cells called neurons. The adult human brain is thought to have between 80 and 100 billion of them. Neurons consist of a main cell body and a long, slender extension known as an axon (Fig. 4.1).

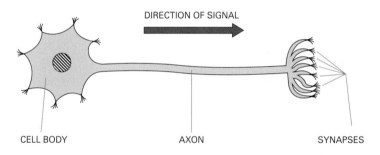

DIRECTION OF SIGNAL

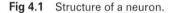

CELL BODY　　　　　　　　AXON　　　　　　　　SYNAPSES

Fig 4.1 Structure of a neuron.

When stimulated, the neuron cell body produces an electrical signal that passes down the long axon at a speed of up to 250 miles per hour. At the end of the axon, the nerve cell opens out into several branching arms which can connect to other neurons, like a link in a chain (Fig. 4.2).

The electrical signal can be passed along this 'chain' of neurons. Chains of neurons join together to form complex linking systems, known as neural networks. Signals transmitted across these neural networks are, in effect, electrical conversations between different parts of the brain. This is how the brain thinks.

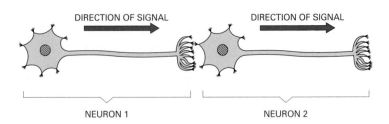

Fig 4.2   Neurons joining up to form a chain.

The synapse

Neurons need to quickly and easily transmit electrical signals between each other. This transmission happens where two neurons meet and this point of contact is known as a synapse (Fig. 4.3). Understanding the synapse is key to understanding how drugs affect the brain because it is here, at the synapse, that most psychoactive drugs work.

Although synapses are the point at which one neuron meets another, the neurons don't actually touch. Instead, there is a very small gap, estimated to be around 20 nanometres wide (that's 0.000002 cm). The electrical signal passes down the axon of the first neuron and reaches the synapse, but isn't able

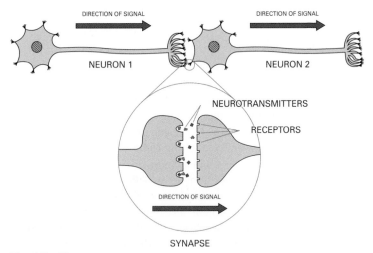

Fig. 4.3   The synapse.

to jump the gap between the first and second neuron. The neuron has to find another way to pass its message on to the next neuron. This mechanism, it turns out, is not electrical but chemical.

The small gap between neurons is crossed when the first neuron releases a small amount of a chemical into the synapse. When used to communicate between neurons, these chemicals are called neurotransmitters. The neurotransmitter moves across the tiny gap to reach the second neuron and attaches to specific sites known as receptors. There are many different types of neurotransmitters and each one has its own corresponding receptor into which only it can fit, like a key fitting into a lock (Fig. 4.4).

NEUROTRANSMITTERS

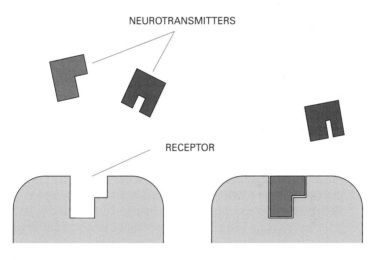

RECEPTOR

Fig. 4.4 Each neurotransmitter has its own unique receptor.

The signal has now been successfully passed from the first neuron to the second. The locking of the neurotransmitter into its receptor causes the second neuron to produce its own, new, electrical signal. This electrical signal then passes down the second neuron until it reaches the end of that neuron and another synapse joining to a third neuron. In this way an electrical signal can be 'passed' along a chain of neurons at very high speed.

Changing the signal strength

Some neurotransmitters increase the likelihood of the second neuron making an electrical signal. They amplify the signal strength, as though turning up the volume. These are called excitatory neurotransmitters. Other neurotransmitters actually reduce the likelihood of the second neuron generating an electrical signal. They muffle the signal, as though turning down the volume. These are called inhibitory neurotransmitters.

Stop or go? How synapses act in complex networks

Neural networks are not just single long chains of neurons. They often involve complex junctions of several neurons meeting at a single synapse. The synapse, through the action of the excitatory and inhibitory neurotransmitters, can act as a 'stop' or 'go' junction for the electrical signal. This stop/go effect, when applied across neural networks with huge numbers of neurons, can work to amplify or diminish activity across the whole network.

What are neural networks used for?

Neural networks are crucial for us to live. The brain continuously communicates vast amounts of information, but most of this signalling happens without our awareness. Many bodily functions, such as our heart beating or our lungs inflating and deflating, happen without us consciously thinking about it. Even complex experiences, such as changes in our mood or level of alertness, can seem to happen without us thinking about them. But actually, complex brain signalling is responsible.

The most complex signalling processes relate to conscious thought and typically involve many different parts of the brain working together. Chapter 2 discussed decision-making and impulsivity and how this affects drug use.

Key messages

- Information travels through the brain as electrical signals along a complex network of interconnecting nerve cells called neurons.
- Neurons connect to each other at synapses, where chemicals called neurotransmitters amplify or muffle the electrical signals.

The brain, pleasure and drugs

Psychoactive drugs change mood, thinking, consciousness and behaviour by hijacking the brain's signalling system. This usually takes place at the synapse, where a drug alters the brain's messaging by increasing or decreasing the strength of the neuronal signal.

Not all psychoactive drugs work in the same way and the exact mechanisms are complex. Some drugs work by mimicking the brain's neurotransmitters and attaching directly to the brain's receptors. Others artificially increase the amount of natural neurotransmitter in the synapse. Both mechanisms exaggerate what goes on in the synapse, changing the signal strength.

Some drugs stimulate and excite the brain (e.g. cocaine, amphetamines). Others sedate it (e.g. cannabis, heroin). Table 4.1 lists the main neurotransmitters, their function in the brain and the common drugs that affect them. By using the brain's existing signalling system to change the way we feel, drugs disturb the balance and function of neurotransmitters and receptors. This can have both immediate and longer-lasting effects.

Table 4.1 Neurotransmitters and the drugs that affect them

Neurotransmitter	Function in the brain	Drugs that affect it
Dopamine	Pleasure, reward	Stimulants (e.g. cocaine, amphetamines)
Serotonin	Mood, sleep, libido, appetite	Ecstasy, LSD, cocaine
Noradrenaline	Sleep, mood, anxiety, memory	Stimulants (e.g. cocaine, amphetamines)
Opioid	Sedation, pain relief, mood	Opioid drugs (e.g. heroin, morphine) and prescribed drugs (e.g. codeine, oxycodone)
Cannabinoid	Cognition, memory, movement	Natural cannabis and synthetic cannabinoids
Glutamate	Learning, cognition, memory	Ketamine, alcohol
Gamma-aminobutyric acid (GABA)	Anxiety, memory, anaesthesia	Sedatives (e.g. benzodiazepines, GHB/GBL) and alcohol

Reward pathways

One particular neural network, sometimes called the 'reward pathway', is responsible for desire and pleasure. It is made up of a chain of neurons that reaches across different parts of the brain. The reward pathway begins deep in the brain and leads to the frontal lobes, the part of the brain where we 'think'. Frontal lobes translate the messages from the reward pathway into conscious feelings of desire, well-being and pleasure.

Dopamine is the main neurotransmitter used by the reward pathway. It's a 'feel good', excitatory neurotransmitter. The reward pathway is very important because it strongly influences how we behave. We tend to repeat behaviours that are pleasurable.

So what makes the brain release dopamine into the reward pathway, and which behaviours cause our brain to signal pleasure? Eating when we are hungry or drinking a glass of water when we are thirsty will stimulate the reward pathway. This in turn makes us feel good and encourages us to continue eating or drinking. Nurturing activities such as cuddling babies also trigger the reward pathway, as do other important behaviours, such as having sex. These activities are not only good for us, they are essential to the survival of the individual and the species. Our brain rewards us for such behaviours by making us feel good.

Too much of a good thing? How the brain regulates pleasure

As attractive as it sounds, we would struggle to function in a state of constant pleasure. The reward pathway not only helps us repeat certain behaviours by making us feel pleasure when we perform them, it also tells us when we have had enough. It does this by shutting off the pleasure before we have too much of a good thing. When we have eaten until full or drunk enough water, dopamine stops being released and the good feelings switch off. Our brain is telling us it is time to stop.

The brain has a good reserve of dopamine, and as long as dopamine is only released in modest amounts, it is easily replenished and the reward system stays in balance.

The reward system and psychoactive drugs

Many psychoactive drugs work by stimulating the reward pathway. By artificially stimulating this pathway, the user can experience very intense pleasure and euphoria. To do this, drugs release much larger amounts of dopamine than would happen with normal behaviours such as eating a delicious meal when hungry.

A stimulant, like cocaine, floods the dopamine receptors with dopamine, 'supercharging' the reward pathway and leading to a very powerful euphoric state. This is what cocaine users call a high. Although very intense, the euphoria usually only lasts a short time. The peak of a cocaine high may only last a few minutes, before receding. This is how a patient, Freddie, described using cocaine.

Freddie's story

Freddie is a 21-year-old man living with his girlfriend in London. He is meeting with me at the request of his employer after he tested positive for cocaine at his annual workplace medical check-up.

Freddie arrives on time and is smartly dressed in a suit and tie. He speaks confidently about his career in the financial district in London, which he greatly enjoys. He works very long hours in the office and also entertains business clients three or four nights a week. Freddie uses cocaine once a week, usually at the weekend, and describes this as his way of rewarding himself for working so hard. He typically snorts 'a few lines' with friends on nights out and has done this since he went to university.

Cocaine gives him 'huge amounts' of energy, makes him feel confident and extremely sociable. He describes an 'unbelievable high', feelings of being powerful and invincible, and huge sexual energy. Freddie also finds that cocaine allows him to drink much more alcohol without feeling intoxicated or tired. He likes drinking alcohol when he uses cocaine because cocaine on its own sometimes makes Freddie's heart race and gives him a feeling of anxiety and panic. The alcohol dampens these feelings and Freddie feels the 'good' effects of cocaine without the 'hassle'.

He admits that there are downsides to using cocaine, including being uncharacteristically aggressive and sexually promiscuous while intoxicated. He is always regretful about his behaviours the following day and comments, 'with cocaine, it always seems to get a bit crazy'. He also experiences a 'come down', which lasts about 24 hours, the day after using cocaine. During this period he feels exhausted and irritable, and has poor concentration and increased anxiety.

The positive drug test came as a shock to Freddie, although he admits that he has been using 'a bit more than usual'. During our session Freddie tells me that he has already decided to stop using cocaine, explaining that although he continues to 'work hard and play hard', he is not going to put his career at risk for something he knows he can do without.

We worked together over four meetings, focusing on strategies to support him to maintain his abstinence from cocaine. He called me a month after our last session to tell me all is going well.

What goes up, must come down

Freddie has described the powerful effects of cocaine. It stimulated his dopamine receptors far beyond normal levels to achieve the euphoria he desired. But in doing so, it disrupted the brain's finely balanced reward system. After the initial, powerful high, the brain needs time to recover and re-establish equilibrium. Freddie's reward pathway shut down during this period, so he felt low in mood, with poor concentration, anxiety and lethargy. Users describe this as a crash or come down, and the feelings don't improve until the brain has recovered. Put simply, you can't have the high without a following low (Fig. 4.5). Table 4.2 describes the short-term (immediately after ingestion) and longer-term (a few days later) effects of cocaine.

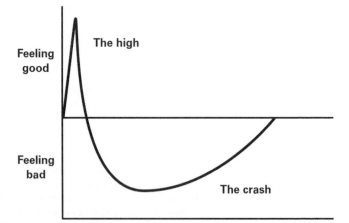

Fig. 4.5 A drug-induced high is generally followed by a 'crash' immediately afterwards.

Table 4.2 Short-term desired and unwanted effects of cocaine

Desired effects		Unwanted effects	
While intoxicated	**Days after use**	**While intoxicated**	**Days after use**
Euphoria	None	Anxiety	Exhaustion
Reduced fatigue		Insomnia	Restlessness
Decreased appetite		Severe headache	Agitation
Increased sex drive		Jaw clenching	Insomnia
Increased ability to concentrate on tasks		Paranoia and psychosis	Irritability
Decreased need for sleep		Irritability, aggression, occasionally violence	
Increased energy and alertness		Racing heart, palpitations, chest pain, occasionally heart attack	
		Dramatically increased blood pressure, occasionally stroke	
		Confusion	
		Seizures	

What happens if you keep on using cocaine?

If someone uses cocaine occasionally, the euphoria is followed by a period of unwanted symptoms as the brain recovers. It takes time to reset the reward pathway after the over-stimulation. But what if cocaine is used again before the brain has recovered?

Regular cocaine use causes the brain to change. The reward pathway doesn't have time to recover and instead begins to adapt to the repeated over-stimulation. To cope with regular cocaine use, the receptors become less sensitive to the dopamine neurotransmitter. In effect, the brain turns down the volume of the reward pathway.

Users experience these changes as a 'wearing off' of the cocaine effect. Regular cocaine use will simply not give the same high for very long. This process is described as tolerance. The brain has changed to cope with the repeated cocaine use by making itself less sensitive to cocaine. For most psychoactive drugs, the more frequently they are used, the greater the likelihood of tolerance. As we will see later, tolerance is an important feature of addiction.

What happens to 'normal' pleasure?

For the drug user, no experience is as intensely rewarding as the drug. Normal experiences just can't compete. The sun on your face sitting in the park, a wonderful meal with friends or listening to an uplifting piece of music – things that would usually result in joy no longer compare to the artificial high of the drug of choice. As the reward pathway adapts to cope with repeated drug use, normal pleasures get caught up in the changes. Tolerance affects both drug-induced and normal pleasure. Drug effects are artificial and unsustainable, but they also wipe out normal pleasures along the way. Regular drug users eventually experience the world as flat, empty, joyless and pointless (Fig. 4.6).

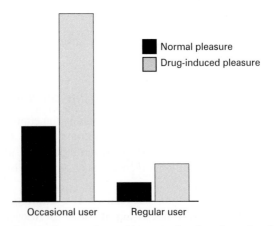

Fig. 4.6 How pleasure is experienced by occasional and regular drug users.

Roger's story

Roger is 22 years old. He works part-time as a fireman and loves his job. He has been a fireman for 2 years and is known on his team for being the strongest and fittest at the station when it comes to lifting and assembling equipment. Roger is passionate about the gym, which he attends at least five times a week.

Roger first tried drugs when he was 15 years old, smoking a few joints of cannabis. Not liking the feeling of being out of control, he stopped. If asked, Roger would say he didn't mind people using drugs but that they were not for him. He drinks alcohol only very occasionally, as it interferes with his exercise programme at the gym.

Six months ago, Roger was at a friend's birthday and, unusually for him, had drunk alcohol. He was really enjoying himself when a close friend offered him cocaine. Perhaps because he was a little drunk, he said yes with minimal persuasion. He only took a very small amount, a fraction of a gram, but experienced an overwhelming feeling of euphoria and well-being unlike anything he had ever known. He felt sociable, full of confidence and with seemingly unlimited energy. Although people had always enjoyed Roger's company, he now felt at the centre of the party and the wittiest person in the room. He felt that people were laughing hysterically at his jokes and he enjoyed their attention. He also found that night that he was able to drink alcohol excessively without feeling even slightly intoxicated. Roger woke the next morning and was surprised that he felt 'great'. He didn't seek out any further cocaine, but a few months later he was offered it by the same friend. Roger accepted and described having another 'magic' night.

After the second time, Roger began to seek out cocaine every few weeks, and continued to enjoy it. He did not experience any harmful effects and, although he tended to miss the occasional gym session, he felt that cocaine was 'just a bit of fun'. Over the next 6 months, his use slowly escalated and he described the cocaine as sometimes being 'rubbish'. He realised that he was using more often and also now needed 'at least a gram' to achieve the effects he had experienced when he first took cocaine.

Unfortunately, about this time Roger was made redundant and it is still not clear if his drug use played any role in this. He was distraught at losing a job he loved and felt he was good at. His cocaine use at this point increased dramatically to three or four times a week and his pattern changed from using at parties to using at home on his own. Roger was now irritated by his drug use. He felt he was spending more money than he could afford on cocaine that wasn't having the effect it used to have. He began using cocaine in the mornings 'just to get the day started' and was now regularly using 2–3 grams a day, 4–5 days a week, and drinking alcohol on the other days. He had given up his gym membership as it was 'too expensive' but was still able to find money for cocaine.

A few weeks ago, Roger was rushed to hospital with severe chest pain. He told the doctor about his cocaine use. He felt huge relief at finally admitting his problem and, after talking through his options with the doctor, agreed to seek help. The next day he came to the clinic.

Chasing the high

When tolerance develops, there are only two ways to recapture the powerful high experienced with the initial drug use. One way is to stop using the drug and let the reward system recover from the over-use. This takes time. The brain needs to reverse the process of receptor change. Recovery can take weeks or even months.

The second option is to use a larger dose of the drug. In the short term, consuming larger amounts of the drug can briefly increase desired effects such as euphoria, but before long the reward pathways will adapt to the new, higher dose, and the drug effects will again fade.

A gradual increase in the amount of drug consumed is often a forewarning of serious trouble ahead. Over time, drug doses can increase considerably, sometimes resulting in huge quantities being used. Doses that would have easily killed the user, if taken when they first started using drugs, now have only minimal effect due to tolerance.

My patients often describe this process as 'chasing the high'. They nostalgically talk about their early drug use as an unforgettably intense experience that they have never really managed to recreate, despite using larger and larger quantities of the drug. They are describing the brain changes of tolerance.

There will come a point when the reward system stops working altogether. When this happens, users don't experience the euphoric high any more, however much of the drug they take. However, although high doses may not produce euphoria any more, they can and often do cause harm such as stroke, heart attack, dependence, depression and psychosis. The desired effects have faded but the risks keep increasing.

Why would someone continue to use a psychoactive drug when it has stopped working and the dangers have increased? Chasing the high is one reason, but other reasons include preventing withdrawal symptoms, wishing to remain part of a particular peer group and even just seeking a feeling of normality.

Key messages

- The reward pathway determines our experience of pleasure and many psychoactive drugs work by over-stimulating this pathway.

- After using psychoactive drugs, the brain needs time to recover. This is often experienced as a psychological 'crash' or 'come down'.

- If a drug is used regularly, the desired effects become harder to achieve – a process called tolerance.

- Users often increase the amount of drug they take over time in an attempt to overcome tolerance. This increases the risk of drug-related harm.

- Regular psychoactive drug users end up altering their brain functioning, making it much harder to enjoy non-drug experiences. The world becomes joyless.

How do drugs cause harm?

Drugs are usually short acting – their effects last anything from a few minutes to a few hours. So why do they cause problems and how? The concept of harm is complex as it can relate to different things. The harm a drug causes a person can be:

- physical (e.g. heart problems)
- psychological (e.g. depression)
- social (e.g. affecting school performance).

Some harm is specific to particular drugs. For example, ketamine can damage the bladder. Other harm relates to the impact of drug use in general.

Harms from drug use don't just happen to the person using the drug but can affect other people too. Damage to relationships with family and friends, road traffic accidents while intoxicated, and involvement in crime are examples of wider harms caused by drug use. Table 4.3 shows the common harm caused by psychoactive drugs.

Table 4.3 Common harm caused by psychoactive drug use

	Harm to the individual (short-term)	Harm to the individual (longer-term)	Harm to others
Physical	Overdose, collapse, confusion, stroke, chest pain, heart problems, vomiting, seizures (fits), lack of coordination, accidents while intoxicated	Insomnia, hepatitis, HIV, lung, kidney, liver, bladder and nerve damage, sexual impotence, vitamin deficiency	Violence
Psychological	Anxiety, panic attack, risk-taking and impaired judgement, losing touch with reality, emotional crash afterwards	Depression, anxiety, mood swings, loss of pleasure, damage to mental functions	Damaged relationships with family and friends
Social	Missing school	Worsening social and academic performance, school expulsion	Crime to fund drug use or while intoxicated

How quickly does harm develop?

Harm can be immediate (acute) or delayed (chronic). A panic attack is an immediate harm associated with stimulants, such as cocaine. The experience is extremely distressing, but usually improves as the drug wears off. Other harms develop with repeated drug use and are sometimes called chronic harms. These harms continue long after the drug has worn off. An example is drug-induced depression.

The speed at which harm develops depends on the individual drug and the way it is used. Some of the harms from cocaine, for example, develop very quickly. The very first time a person uses cocaine, they may experience severe chest pain due to the powerful constricting effect of the drug on the coronary arteries. This can cause a heart attack (Agrawal *et al*, 2015). But other harm is more likely when cocaine is consumed repeatedly over a longer period. Low mood and depression can develop over time, as the brain becomes chronically depleted of dopamine and other neurotransmitters.

How does the harmfulness of different drugs compare?

Some drugs are more harmful than others. Researchers have estimated the relative harmfulness of different drugs by combining the harm to the individual with the harm to others (Nutt *et al*, 2007). By this measure, alcohol, heroin and crack cocaine are the most harmful drugs. Fig. 4.7 shows an estimate of the harm caused by different drugs.

Most harm caused by psychoactive drug use is predictable. However, sometimes drug-related harm occurs that is unexpected and out of proportion with the amount of drug

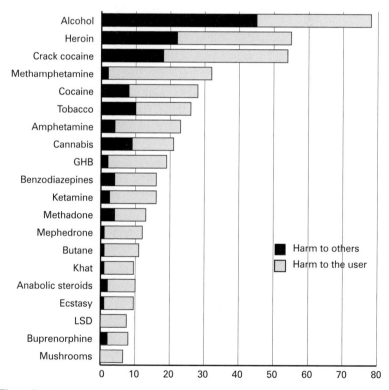

Fig. 4.7 The amount of harm to the user and to others that is caused by different drugs (maximum possible rating is 100). (Adapted with permission from Nutt *et al*, 2010.)

taken. This is called an idiosyncratic drug reaction. Hallucinogen persisting perception disorder (HPPD) is an example.

Arnold's story

Arnold is an 18-year-old university student in his first year of a computer programming degree. He is very committed to his studies and wants to start his own software company developing mobile phone apps. He is popular and seen by his peers as likeable, engaging and extroverted. The first time I meet Arnold, a friend comes with him in support.

When we meet, he is softly spoken and gentle in his manner. He looks nervous and regularly glances at his friend for encouragement. He begins to tell me about himself, explaining that he rarely uses drugs and when he does, which is usually twice a year, he takes ecstasy while clubbing. Arnold has taken seven tablets of ecstasy in his life. His only other drug use, apart from an occasional alcoholic drink, involved smoking a few joints of cannabis when he was 16 years old.

When Arnold took his last ecstasy tablet, he had expected to enjoy the experience as he had done on all of the previous occasions. This time, however, was very different. Within 30 minutes of taking the drug, he experienced frightening 'shadows' at the periphery of his vision, which disappeared when he tried to look at them. He also saw bright, 'streaky' lights flashing across his field of vision. Arnold had never experienced anything like this before and found it very distressing. He told his friends he was not feeling well and went home. On his way back from the club, the visual symptoms continued, but he was able to fall asleep once home. The next morning, his symptoms were still there and he also saw 'fuzziness' around the edges of objects when he looked at them. If he stared at an object, for example a cup on a table in front of him, the object seemed to gradually increase in size before shrinking again. To Arnold, it looked like the cup was breathing.

Arnold rang his friends, who suggested that he had probably taken a 'bad pill' of ecstasy, that things would improve and that he just needed to wait things out.

Over the next few days, Arnold's symptoms showed no sign of improvement and he began to panic, fearing that he had damaged his brain. The shadowy figures at the edge of his vision continued day and night and were intimidating and frightening. He was unable to concentrate on anything.

Eventually, a week after he had taken the ecstasy, Arnold went to see his general practitioner (GP). They agreed that he had probably taken a particularly strong dose or possibly even another drug entirely that had been mis-sold as ecstasy.

The GP gave Arnold a small amount of diazepam and told him to return in a week. The diazepam helped to reduce the intensity of the visual experiences but they did not stop completely. Over the next few weeks the symptoms slowly began to improve. Arnold's GP stopped prescribing diazepam as she was worried that Arnold was at risk of becoming dependent on them.

Two months after taking the ecstasy, Arnold was still experiencing constant symptoms that, although less intense than before, were still very distracting. He was very distressed by the thought that he would never get better and referred himself to see me at the clinic.

The most likely diagnosis is hallucinogen persisting perception disorder, or HPPD. It is a controversial diagnosis that is still poorly defined and some researchers have questioned whether it is real or caused by anxiety (Halpern & Pope, 2003). Symptoms usually resolve on their own, but this can take many months. With long-term symptoms such as Arnold's, it is important to exclude physical causes, such as a small stroke or a brain tumour. We carried out a brain scan, which fortunately was normal.

A psychologist taught Arnold techniques to help him to ignore his symptoms and calm his anxiety, and he found these helpful. He began to feel he was regaining control over the symptoms and felt reassured that they were slowly improving.

I last met Arnold in clinic 5 months after he took the ecstasy. His symptoms had significantly improved. The shadowy figures had gone completely and he only saw occasional faint, 'streaking lights'. He still found his vision to be 'more intense', but this was also improving. I explained that his symptoms were likely to return if he used drugs again. Arnold did not know what dose or even which drug he really consumed that night, but was certain he would never take drugs again.

It is not clear why Arnold experienced these idiosyncratic symptoms, when his friends who took the same batch of ecstasy did not. It could be that he inadvertently consumed a particularly high dose, or that a more harmful drug had been substituted for ecstasy. Arnold might also have an individual vulnerability to psychoactive drugs, making him more likely to experience harm than his peers.

Are some people more vulnerable to drug harm?

Most people agree that smoking cigarettes is harmful because they know smoking causes heart disease, bronchitis and cancer. But most people, particularly smokers, know someone who has smoked without any significant problems. Typically, these stories include an elderly relative who smoked 'like a chimney' all their life and now, in their 90s, is 'as fit as a fiddle'. These examples are often used to describe people who 'got away with it', apparently using a harmful substance for much of their life but without significant problems. They seem to be resistant to the harmful effects that others typically experience. My patients sometimes frustratedly talk about how unfair it is that their friends seem able to use drugs without any apparent problems, while they have ended up needing to see a psychiatrist.

What is clear is that people have different vulnerabilities to drug harm. Two people can consume exactly the same amount of a drug and experience different desired effects and also different harmful effects. This is crucial information. If you knew in advance that you were particularly vulnerable to a drug, you probably wouldn't take it. Imagine you know that you are particularly at risk of suffering a cocaine-induced heart attack. Would you avoid cocaine at all costs? Many people probably would.

So what determines individual vulnerability to drugs and how can we predict whether a particular person is at greater risk? Calculating a person's risk is complex and there are several things to think about. These can be divided into two broad groups:

- the drug itself
  - the type of drug
  - the way the drug is taken
  - the amount taken
  - how long the drug is taken for
- the person taking the drug
  - genetic make-up
  - emotional health
  - physical health
  - social health.

Let's look at each of these in turn.

Drug-related factors

The type of drug

Some drugs are more powerful in their effects, causing greater changes in the brain. Cocaine is a more powerful stimulant than caffeine, and heroin is a more powerful depressant than codeine. A drug's power, or potency as it is technically called, usually relates to the strength of drug's effect on the synapses in the brain. Potency is important, as it tends to correlate closely to the likelihood of harm.

How the drug is used

Drugs come in a variety of forms, such as powders, pills, liquids, gases and solutions, and can be consumed in many ways, such as by smoking, snorting or swallowing it, dissolving it in a drink, injecting it, placing it against the gums, inhaling it, and taking it rectally. The way a drug is consumed has a huge impact on how quickly it reaches the brain, which partially determines its effect.

If a drug is smoked or injected, it reaches the brain very quickly. This leads to a rapid, powerful effect, but one that is often relatively short-lasting. Taking a drug as a pill or drink means the drug needs to be absorbed from the stomach and intestines before it can reach the brain. This takes longer and results in a less intense, slower but longer-lasting effect. Fig. 4.8 compares the effects of swallowing or injecting drugs.

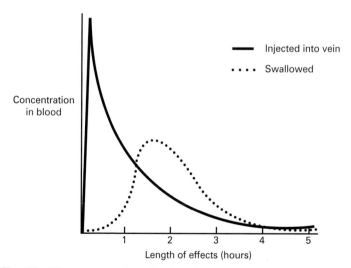

Fig. 4.8 The concentration of a drug in the blood and the length of its effects when swallowed or injected.

Generally, the most harmful way of taking a drug is by injection. People who inject drugs tend to experience the worst harm and have the poorest response to treatment of all drug users. Injecting is also the most risky way to take a drug. The amount of drug taken by injection can easily be misjudged. Instead of a rapid, intense high, the user can take too much and overdose. Other harms from injecting result from the act of injecting itself – for example, skin infections or the transmission of blood-borne viruses such as hepatitis and HIV.

The amount of drug taken (dose)

The concept of dose is familiar to us from prescribed medication. An antibiotic prescription might say something like 'one capsule, three times a day, for five days'. The prescription tells us precisely how much of the drug to take (one capsule), how often (three times a day) and for how long (five days). For other medications, there is no fixed dosing regimen, instead the medication is taken only when the symptoms are present. Think of a headache: you might adjust the amount of painkiller you take, perhaps taking one tablet first, and only if your headache continues would you take a second dose a few hours later.

We can apply the concept of dose to psychoactive drugs. Typically, the more you consume, the larger the effect. Two 'lines' of cocaine should in theory cause greater euphoria than one line. There are big differences however between medications and illicit psychoactive drugs. One of these differences relates to their manufacture.

Commercial medications, such as antibiotics or painkillers, are produced to very strict standards with clear regulation and quality assurance. Each dose, whether it is a tablet, syrup or powder,m has to be carefully manufactured so that it has the correct quantity of drug. The drug itself will only be one part of a medicine and other inactive ingredients are used to make up the rest. These inactive ingredients are also carefully regulated and controlled. Futhermore, medications are manufactured in laboratories with strict rules regarding hygiene and cleanliness, to avoid any contamination.

By contrast, illicit drug manufacture is completely unregulated. There is nobody checking to see whether the product is safe, reliable or of the correct quality. Occasionally this results in disaster, as when a batch of heroin sold in Scotland in 2009/2010 became accidentally infected with anthrax leading to 47 users becoming infected and 14 dying (National Anthrax Outbreak Control Team, 2011).

As well as accidental contamination through poor standards of production, another effect of unregulated production is huge differences in strength or potency. This variation in strength means that the user has no way of judging the likely effect of the drug. It could be very strong or very weak, but the user won't know until the drug is in their body, by which time it is too late to do anything about it.

Some of this variation in strength comes from poor manufacturing standards. At other times, it is due to deliberate dilution of the drug, a process sometimes called 'cutting' or 'bulking' the drug. These 'cutting' or 'bulking' ingredients increase the apparent quantity or volume of the drug and, of course, increase profit. Unlike regulated pharmaceutical medications, these added substances are not generally safe, harmless ingredients but are instead often a range of potentially hazardous chemicals.

A step beyond this is not just to dilute the drug with inactive ingredients, which may weaken the drug effect, but to add in other, cheaper, psychoactive ingredients to the original drug that can mimic some of the effects anticipated by the user.

In some cases, drugs sold in the illegal market contain none of the stated drug at all. It has either been replaced with a similar, but cheaper and inferior, drug or occasionally it is a complete dud, containing no psychoactive substance. The user is hardly likely to complain to the police that their illegal drugs are not good enough quality!

So although the dose of psychoactive drug is critical to the harm it may cause, many people using illicit drugs have little or no idea what dose, or very often even what drug, they are taking. Once the drug has been taken, there is nothing the user can do about it, even if they realise they don't like the effects it is having on them. This gamble with the dose is a huge risk, particularly for overdose, but is one that many users take without much thought.

How long the drug is used

As mentioned earlier, drug harm can be immediate or develop with repeated drug use. While occasionally people experience extreme harm or even death the very first time they use a psychoactive substance, more commonly the risks increase with repeated use. For most people, the more you take the bigger the risks.

Harms can build up over time, as the brain and other parts of the body struggle to recover from the toxic effects of the drug. Damage to the brain, known as neurotoxicity, causes deterioration in functions such as memory and concentration. Other organs, such as the kidneys, liver and bladder can also be damaged by regular drug use.

Person-related factors

Individuals have different vulnerabilities to both using drugs and experiencing problems. Vulnerability is based on a range of factors that combine to account for an individual's risk. Understanding your personal risk of harm from drugs is critical, because perceived personal risk can affect our choices and behaviour. Some of the most important vulnerabilities include genetic make-up, mental and physical health, and environment.

Drug-related harm and genetics

Some people have a vulnerability to psychoactive drugs written into their genes (Swendsen & Le Moal, 2001). Our genetic code not only determines our physical characteristics (e.g. eye colour), it also influences the pattern and profile of our brain's receptors. These receptors are crucial in determining the way the brain responds to drugs. As a result, some people have brains that are more sensitive to the effects of drugs, both wanted and unwanted. But it is not just vulnerability to the immediate effects of drugs that is individually encoded. Vulnerability to longer-term problems such as becoming physically and psychologically dependent on drugs is also partly determined by our genetic make-up (Swendsen & Le Moal, 2011).

The importance of our genetic make-up seems to differ from drug to drug. Some studies suggest that around a third of the risk of cannabis dependence is genetic (Agrawal & Lynskey, 2006), whereas other studies suggest genetic make-up contributes to half the statistical risk of heroin use (Tsuang *et al*, 1998).

Examining a family tree can help us to understand genetic vulnerability, and a clinical assessment of problematic drug use should include asking if there is a family history of drug use. 'Has anybody in your family experienced problems with alcohol, drugs or gambling?' is a typical screening question.

It is important to remember that having a relative or even several relatives with drug problems does not mean that you or your children will inevitably end up with one. A better way to think about it is that, if you have a family tree containing significant drug problems, you and your children are more vulnerable to having problems. You are at greater risk, and you can't change your genes. You can, however, make decisions based on this knowledge.

Mental health

Using psychoactive drugs can lead to a range of mental health problems, but it can also work the other way round – having a mental health problem can increase the risk of harmful drug use (Glantz *et al*, 2009). Some people take drugs to bring them relief from their existing mental health symptoms, often unintentionally worsening them instead. For example, some stimulant users take drugs to briefly relieve the low energy and sluggish thinking of depression, while some cannabis users say the drug relieves anxiety. However, in both these examples, repeated drug use is likely to worsen the very mental health problems the users are trying to relieve.

Childhood physical, sexual or emotional abuse is associated with an increased risk of early, severe drug use (Moran *et al*, 2004; World Health Organization, 2009). This might be because drugs are used to help manage difficult emotions or mental health problems related to the trauma. Intoxication can offer a tantalising, if brief, period of escape from mental health problems.

Unfortunately, drug use causes much greater problems over time. Using drugs when you already have mental health problems risks exacerbating those problems: worsening low mood, increasing anxiety and heightening psychosis. Worse still, drug users tend to be less engaged with the mental health treatments that tackle these problems. Drug use ends up being doubly harmful, worsening mental health and throwing up barriers to getting help.

Physical health

Physical health problems can also increase the risk of drug use. An example is chronic pain (Action on Addiction, 2013). Psychoactive drugs, particularly strong opioids with powerful pain-reducing effects, can be extremely helpful in reducing pain when prescribed by a health professional in the context of treatment. Problems arise, however, when they are used without medical supervision, as there is a risk that their use can rapidly become uncontrollable. The legitimate medical treatment can become part of the problem.

Social health

Social health refers to a person's level of functioning in their environment and includes a range of interlinked factors, such as family structure, income, occupation, social network, quality of housing and culture. Many of these factors influence the risk of drug use (Marmot *et al*, 2010).

Family life has been shown to be protective against drug use if strong relationships and good communication exist. But family members can increase the risk of their children using drugs if they use drugs themselves, have high levels of conflict with the child and poorly monitor their child's behaviour (McArdle *et al*, 2002).

Peers are also an important influence on the likelihood of drug use. People tend to seek out like-minded friends with shared values, which may include drug use. Alternatively, there may be a pressure to conform by engaging in behaviours, such as drug use, that increase acceptance and allow membership to a particular peer group.

Social health also extends to the surrounding environment. Living in safe, clean housing in an area with little community drug use reduces a person's risk of using drugs. There is a relationship between socioeconomic status and drug use, with greater social deprivation predicting higher levels of drug use (Marmot *et al*, 2010).

> **Key messages**
>
> - Psychoactive drug use can cause physical, psychological and social harm.
> - Drug-related harm depends on factors related to the drug and factors related to the person.
> - Drug-related factors include the type of drug, how it is used, the amount taken and the length of use.
> - Person-related factors include genetic make-up as well as mental, physical and social health.

Addiction and dependence

Addiction and dependence are perhaps the most commonly talked about problems related to psychoactive drug use. It is hard to read the news without finding a story about a celebrity being admitted to rehab for one or more 'addictions'. People also sometimes describe themselves as having an 'addictive personality' because they have just finished off the last of the chocolates or are returning to play one more level of a computer game. The terms 'addiction' and 'addictive personality' are often used by the media as shorthand for impulsivity, a lack of self-discipline and emotional problems.

The popular media concept of addiction has broadened in recent years to include behaviours such as gambling, sex, eating, shopping and even texting. So, what is addiction, how is it different from dependence, and if you use drugs, does it mean you are an addict? Is there such thing as an addictive personality? Can you be addicted to shopping?

Drug dependence is a medical illness

It is now widely accepted by scientists and clinicians that, for some individuals, harmful drug use is not just rebellious behaviour, poor judgement or a lack of willpower. Instead, drug-using behaviour can result from underlying problems in brain function and as such is a treatable medical condition. In these people, the underlying brain problems interact with other factors including family relationships, peer groups and stress to influence drug-using behaviour. For this group, defining their

73

behaviour as a medical condition is important, as it legitimises treatment, just as for any other medical condition.

Given that some people have drug problems because of an underlying brain problem, how can they be identified so that treatment can be offered? The answer lies in a careful assessment of their pattern of drug use.

Patterns of drug use

Accurately describing patterns of drug use helps the clinician understand the extent of the problem and work out if treatment might help. Three terms are commonly used by clinicians to describe the way a drug is used and the impact of that use:

- recreational use
- harmful use
- dependence syndrome.

Recreational use

This term describes drug use that does not cause significant physical, psychological or social harm.

Jackie's story

Jackie is a bright, articulate, 19-year-old university student who hopes to become an English teacher. She is immediately likeable and popular with her peers, who know her for being outgoing, warm and sociable.

Jackie first drank alcohol at a party when she was 15 years old. With no experience of alcohol, she drank far too much and felt very unwell the next day. Because of this experience, she now avoids alcohol if offered, despite many of her peers binge-drinking most weekends.

When Jackie was 16 years old, she was offered cannabis at a party. She accepted and really enjoyed the relaxed and giggly feeling it gave her, much preferring it to alcohol. She was not offered it again and did not seek it out. It was not until Jackie arrived at university that she came across cannabis for a second time. Many of her new friends smoked cannabis and one of them knew a student in the year above who would sell them cannabis whenever they wanted it.

Over the past year, Jackie has smoked cannabis less than 10 times. Each time, she has smoked with friends at parties, except on one occasion when she wanted to see if cannabis improved her creative essay writing (it didn't, as she fell asleep and the essay was handed in late).

Jackie denies any problems with her cannabis use and thinks it is fun to smoke it 'now and again'. She is now careful not to use cannabis if she has assignments to hand in and does not think her use has affected her academic studies at all. If her friend was no longer able to buy cannabis, Jackie does not think she would try and buy it herself because she is worried about 'mixing with the wrong people' and getting caught. Jackie plans to stop using cannabis after university, as she wants to get a teaching job. She thinks it would be unacceptable to be using cannabis once she is a teacher but for now sees her drug use as part of student life.

Harmful use

Harmful use is defined by the World Health Organization (2015a) as a pattern of drug use 'that is causing damage to health'. The damage may be physical or mental. This is a broad definition that can include a wide range of different harms, but the key element is that the drug user has moved on from recreational use and is now harming themself.

Greg's story

Greg is a 16-year-old schoolboy due to sit exams this year and hoping to study music at university. Greg has been interested in music for as long as he can remember and particularly likes electronic dance music. He has set up a small recording studio in his bedroom and records music that he sells to his friends. He also does some DJ-ing at friends' parties and was recently paid to DJ at an event run at a local social club. Greg believes that to DJ well he needs to be 'in the moment' and has experimented with drugs to help him achieve this. He began with ecstasy but found it too stimulating. On two occasions he felt his heart racing at 'a hundred miles an hour' and was so sure that he was having a heart attack that he stopped DJ-ing to go home to rest.

More recently, Greg has tried ketamine. He believes small doses improve his music-making and he has started using ketamine whenever he DJs, which is most weekends. In the past month, Greg has found ketamine increasingly 'more-ish' and has begun to take it during the week when he is making music at home in his room.

A week ago, Greg noticed that his urine had turned dark brown and he felt an intense pain across his lower abdomen. He had experienced some mild lower abdominal pain for the past few weeks that he assumed was a muscle strain. Alarmed, he went to see his GP, thinking that he may have a urine infection. The tests showed no infection but did reveal blood in his urine. It was not until he told one of his friends about his symptoms that they explained that he probably had 'ketamine bladder'.

Ketamine can severely damage the inner lining of the bladder, causing ulceration, bleeding into the urine, pain on urination and lower abdominal pain. Ketamine-related bladder damage only tends to occur when people use ketamine regularly and some heavy ketamine users damage their bladders so severely that they need surgical repair or even bladder removal.

Greg was shocked by this information and stopped using ketamine immediately. Fortunately, his symptoms completely resolved within a few weeks. He continues to DJ but has made a decision to use drugs only on 'special occasions'.

Dependence syndrome

Dependence syndrome is a term defined by the WHO (2015b) and describes a pattern of drug use that, over time, leads to the following features.

- An overwhelming and uncontrollable **desire to use** the drug.
- A **loss of control** over how much of the drug is consumed.
- **Tolerance** to the effect of the drug, resulting in the user needing larger and larger amounts of the drug to achieve the same effect.
- Physical **withdrawal symptoms** if the drug use is reduced or stopped.
- A loss of interest in other activities. Using the **drug becomes more important** than anything else.
- **Continuing to use** the drug even when it is clearly causing harm.

Three or more of the above features need to be present in the past year to fulfil the criteria for dependence syndrome.

Andy's story

Andy is a 19-year-old man living with friends and working as a shop manager. He has been using cannabis, ecstasy and alcohol since he was 14 years old but always with friends and only every few weeks. After starting work, Andy stopped using drugs but continued to binge on alcohol most Friday and Saturday nights with friends in the pub. A year ago, a friend of a friend introduced Andy to cocaine. For Andy, this was the most amazing drug he had ever tried. He found it mixed very well with alcohol, allowing him to drink much more than he could possibly have managed without cocaine.

He also liked the way he felt, as the cocaine made him highly sociable, euphoric and full of energy.

Andy began to use cocaine 'once in a while', but after a few months noticed that his consumption had increased to most weekends and that he was spending more money than he could really afford on the drug. He decided to stop using cocaine for a few weeks, but the very next weekend used more cocaine than ever before, spending nearly £300 in two days on cocaine and alcohol. Andy was late for work the following Monday as he 'felt like death'. He told his boss he had flu and went home to bed. He was annoyed with himself and also surprised at his lack of control. Andy spoke to his housemates and they agreed it was time to 'calm it down'.

However, on the next weekend the same thing happened. Andy used far more cocaine than he intended to use on Friday and Saturday night and spent all of Sunday recovering. The following week he felt anxious, tearful and sad. He promised himself that he would take a break from the cocaine, as he recognised that it was now causing him problems.

The following weekend, Andy stayed in on Friday night but spent all evening thinking about cocaine and regretting that he was 'missing out'. By the following evening, he had returned to cocaine, unable to resist his powerful impulse to use. He described having a 'brilliant' night but admitted using 'ridiculous' amounts of cocaine. Andy's friends began to worry about him, as did his boss at work.

Andy's cocaine use began to spiral out of control. He started using during the week as well as every weekend. He ran up a debt with his cocaine dealer, who was only too happy to offer credit and continue supplying the drug. After two formal warnings for excessive absences, Andy's boss sacked him.

Andy began using cocaine every day, on his own rather than with friends. He had become tolerant to the effects of the drug and no longer experienced any euphoria at all. Instead, using cocaine only helped to take away his severe cravings and help him 'get out of bed, be up and about and functioning'. When not using cocaine, he felt very depressed and anxious and on two occasions had thoughts of suicide. His dealer started physically threatening Andy, insisting that he repay the money he owed. Andy had stopped going out except to buy cocaine.

Finally, one of Andy's friends contacted his parents, who arranged for him to come to the clinic. During assessment, as he began to tell his story, he realised how uncontrollable his life had become. Andy recognised that he could no longer help himself and agreed to start treatment. Following a medically assisted detoxification from cocaine, Andy went to a residential rehabilitation programme where he learned the psychological skills to live life without cocaine or other drugs. On leaving the residential programme, he attended Cocaine Anonymous, which he found very supportive. He has so far avoided any relapses and is looking for work, but admits that he is still taking things one day at a time.

Patterns of use, consequences and treatment

The pattern of use and the subsequent consequences are different in these three case studies. Most drug users fall in the recreational group and, like Jackie, use drugs for a while but reduce or stop using, depending on their circumstances. But some recreational users progress to harmful use, like Greg. Relatively few develop dependence, as Andy did with cocaine, but this group experiences the most harm and has the most need of help.

The useful thing about describing drug use in terms of whether it is recreational, harmful or dependent is that it doesn't matter what drug or drugs someone is using. Instead, it is the pattern of use that helps clinicians understand the extent of the problem and identify the best treatment. Matching treatment to the problem is important and will be discussed in Chapter 8.

What about addiction?

Addiction is a popular term and one that is widely used in the media. It is not often used by clinicians because it is poorly defined. Perhaps the best way to think about addiction is to consider it as similar to dependence syndrome, but with the difference that addiction includes both harm to the person using the drug and wider harm to those around them.

Is there such thing as an addictive personality?

I frequently hear people describe themselves as having an 'addictive personality'. People generally use this expression when they find it difficult to say no to things, for example alcohol, drugs or food. It is also sometimes used to describe an intense drive or compulsion to engage in activities beyond the point where most people would stop.

One of the problems with the concept of an addictive personality is that it is used to describe such a wide range of people and issues: from people who can't stop until they have finished a tub of ice cream to those who experience a thrill from extreme sports. The term is so broad that it is unhelpful.

Research has yet to reveal a clearly definable addictive personality. However, there are characteristics or traits that increase the risk of drug use: impulsivity (engaging in behaviour without adequate thought about the consequences) and sensation-seeking. These two personality traits are linked to poor decision-making in general and drug use in particular (Staiger *et al*, 2007). Chapter 2 looked at the developing adolescent brain and why impulsivity and sensation-seeking peak at this age.

There is also a 'chicken and egg' dilemma to consider when thinking about addictive personality and drug use. Although some personality traits increase the risk of using drugs, using drugs can also change the personality, particularly during adolescence when the brain is rapidly developing and vulnerable to damage from drugs. Persistent negative thinking, irritability and social withdrawal have all been identified as personality changes that can develop when drugs are used. It is often hard to untangle whether a person's personality led them to use drugs or whether the drug use itself damaged their brain.

Behavioural addiction: can you be addicted without a drug?

Research is now showing that some behaviour can follow similar harmful patterns as those seen in drug use. The most widely accepted is gambling (Leeman & Potenza, 2012). Pathological gamblers describe difficulty controlling their level of use, an overpowering compulsion to gamble even when they know that they do not have the funds, and a loss of interest in other activities. They also describe other features seen in drug dependence, such as the gradual escalation of use and continued use despite clear harm to themselves and others.

The thrill a pathological gambler experiences when gambling has been shown to cause changes in the brain that are similar to those caused by some drugs. Many of the changes in thinking seen in drug dependence, such as poor decision-making and emotional processing, are also seen in pathological gamblers.

There is less evidence for other behavioural addictions, but researchers are currently exploring whether activities such as excessive video-game playing or use of pornography share the same underlying brain mechanisms as drug dependence.

Key messages

- Drug use can be broadly classified as recreational use, harmful use or dependence syndrome.
- Drug dependence is a medical condition resulting from faulty brain functioning.
- Understanding patterns of use helps clinicians decide if treatment is needed and, if so, which treatment is most likely to help.
- Some behaviour, such as gambling, can cause brain changes similar to those seen in drug dependence.

Types of drugs

To have a meaningful conversation with your child about drugs, you need to be confident that you have enough information about the different drugs, how they're used, what effects they cause and the risks they carry. This chapter will focus on the key knowledge you need in order to plan the drug conversation.

Psychoactive drugs cause their dramatic effects by influencing the messaging between nerves in the brain. Different drugs work through different receptors to cause particular effects on feelings and behaviours. A strong cup of coffee makes us feel alert and energised, whereas too much alcohol makes us feel sleepy and tired. This is because caffeine works by stimulating the brain, whereas alcohol causes sedation. Knowing the types of drugs is important, because it helps us understand the risks associated with them.

You will have heard of some drugs, for example heroin, cocaine or cannabis. But in addition to these well-known drugs, there are hundreds of more obscure drugs available, sometimes better known by their brand names.

Psychoactive drugs can be broadly classified into four groups according to their primary effect:

- stimulating
- sedating
- hallucinogenic
- dissociative.

In most cases, the name of a drug gives away little about its probable effects when consumed. Some drugs have more than one effect (Fig. 5.1) or different effects at certain doses. For example, ecstasy (MDMA) has both stimulant and

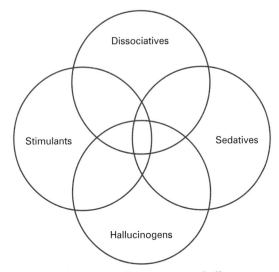

Fig. 5.1 Drugs can have more than one type of effect.

hallucinogenic properties, while ketamine can cause euphoria at lower doses but is sedating at higher doses. Box 5.1 shows the most common drugs within each group.

Key messages

- Psychoactive drugs can be divided into four broad groups according to their effect.
- Stimulants, such as cocaine, cause euphoria and alertness.
- Sedatives, such as cannabis, cause relaxation and calm.
- Hallucinogens, such as LSD, cause hallucinations.
- Dissociatives, such as ketamine, cause 'out-of-body' experiences.

Stimulants

What are stimulant drugs?

As the name suggests, stimulant drugs cause a person to feel alert and energetic, increase concentration and reduce fatigue. Stimulants can also produce powerful feelings of euphoria and well-being. As well as their psychoactive effects, stimulants can

> **Box 5.1**   The most common drugs categorised by psychoactive effect
>
> *Stimulants*
>
> - Cocaine
> - Amphetamine
> - Methamphetamine (crystal meth)
> - Ecstasy
> - Synthetic stimulants
>
> *Sedatives*
>
> - Natural and synthetic cannabis
> - Opioids (e.g. heroin, morphine, codeine)
> - Benzodiazepines
> - GHB/GBL
>
> *Hallucinogens*
>
> - LSD
> - Magic mushrooms
> - Synthetic hallucinogens
>
> *Dissociatives*
>
> - Ketamine
> - Nitrous oxide

produce powerful physical effects, such as a racing heart rate, increased blood pressure and a reduced need to sleep and eat.

Caffeine is a good example of a legal and culturally acceptable stimulant. Those of us who like a strong coffee first thing in the morning will be familiar with the lift in energy, increased alertness and improved concentration it brings. But coffee can also have unwanted effects. Drinking too much can trigger an unpleasant feeling of restlessness, disrupt our sleep and even cause palpitations (feeling your heart beating in your chest).

Other stimulant drugs, such as cocaine and amphetamines, produce much stronger effects. As well as increased alertness, these drugs cause a powerful feeling of euphoria (intense excitement and happiness). The euphoria can be overwhelming and is often called a 'high'. For many users, this is the main attraction of using stimulant drugs. The intense, euphoric high is, for most, well beyond anything they experience in daily life. Common stimulant drugs and their negative effects are listed in Table 5.1.

Table 5.1 Common stimulant drugs and their associated problems

Drug/drug group	Description	Common names[a]	Short-term problems	Long-term problems
Amphetamines	• Synthetic drugs produced in a range of forms including tablets, powders, pastes and solutions • Usually swallowed, snorted or injected	Speed, whizz	Agitation, aggression, racing heart, palpitations, high blood pressure, irregular heart rate, chest pain, heart attack, stroke, confusion, psychosis	Insomnia, depression, anxiety, memory problems, skin-picking, persecutory thinking, psychosis, personality change, tolerance, severe dependence, withdrawal symptoms
Methamphetamine	• Powerful synthetic drug from amphetamine group • Can be swallowed as pills, snorted as powder, smoked as crystals or injected	Crystal meth, crystal, tina, meth	As for amphetamines, but may cause more acute psychosis and risk-taking	As for amphetamines, also severe and rapid dependence
Cocaine (powder)	• Powerful, fast-acting stimulant derived from coca leaves • Local pain-relieving effect • Usually snorted, can be injected	Coke, blow, Charlie	As for amphetamines, but may cause more severe heart problems	As for amphetamines, also nose bleeds with repeated snorting
Cocaine (crack)	• Smokable and injectable version of cocaine made by heating cocaine powder with baking soda (freebasing) • Usually smoked or injected	Crack (the individual crystals are often called rocks or stones)	As for amphetamines	As for amphetamines, also lung problems associated with smoking ('crack lung')
Prescribed stimulants	• Medications used for the treatment of attention-deficit hyperactivity disorder (ADHD) and narcolepsy	Ritalin®, Concerta®, Adderall®, Dexedrine®	As for amphetamines	As for amphetamines

Drug/drug group	Description	Common names[a]	Short-term problems	Long-term problems
Ecstasy (MDMA)	• Synthetic drug popular in electronic dance music settings • Usually swallowed as tablet, snorted as crystalline powder, or 'bombed'/'parachuted' as powder wrapped in paper	Tablets usually referred to as ecstasy, E or molly; powder called MDMA or MD	Nausea, agitation, vomiting, headache, loss of coordination, teeth-grinding and facial 'gurning', insomnia, hallucinations, confusion, psychosis, overheating, swelling of the brain, serotonergic syndrome	Depression, anxiety, memory problems, liver problems, no clear evidence of dependence or withdrawal
Other synthetic stimulants (including cathinones, phenethylamines, tryptamines, piperazines)	• Synthetic stimulants produced to mimic the effects of traditional drugs such as cocaine or ecstasy • Sold online or in head shops • Produced as pills, capsules or powder in foil packets • Usually swallowed or snorted but sometimes injected • The most common in the UK is mephedrone (drone, M-Cat)	Legal highs, research chemicals, drone, M-Cat, meph (huge number of brand names like Gogaine and Benzofury)	As for amphetamines	As for amphetamines
Khat	• Fresh leaves of a shrub grown in East Africa and Arabia • Causes stimulant effects similar to those of amphetamine	Khat	As for amphetamines	As for amphetamines, also probably causes dependence in some users

a. The terms used for drugs differ over time and from place to place. The examples given were common at the time of writing.
Sources: www.drugscope.org.uk and Royal Society for the Encouragement of Arts, Manufactures and Commerce (2007).

How are they used?

Stimulant drugs are easily absorbed by the body and are produced and marketed in a variety of preparations, including powders, tablets and solutions. They can be snorted, swallowed, smoked, injected, applied to the gums ('dabbing') or inserted rectally. Some stimulant drugs can be wrapped in cigarette paper and swallowed, a practice known as 'bombing' or 'parachuting'. In the case of the stimulant plant khat, the leaves are chewed.

What problems can stimulant drugs cause?

Immediate and short-term problems

Stimulants can cause extreme agitation and aggression. They powerfully affect the heart, increasing heart rate and blood pressure and risking irregular heartbeat, chest pain, heart attack and stroke. Stimulant drugs can also cause overheating and insomnia.

Stimulant drugs increase the effects of neurotransmitters, particularly dopamine and serotonin. High levels of serotonin can lead to a life-threatening problem called serotonin syndrome, during which the brain becomes poisoned by too much active serotonin. Symptoms include sweating, overheating, tremor, racing heart, confusion, coma and even death. The risks are greater if two serotonin-boosting drugs are taken simultaneously.

If a person takes too much of a drug, it is called an overdose. When this happens, the person can experience confusion, seizures and psychosis (e.g. losing touch with reality, feeling paranoid, experiencing hallucinations).

Cocaine has particularly powerful effects on blood vessels, causing them to tighten and go into spasm. When this happens in the arteries around the heart, it blocks the flow of oxygen-carrying blood, starving the heart of oxygen. This leads to chest pain and, if the arteries don't re-open, to a heart attack. This can happen to people using cocaine from the very first use.

Problems from repeated use

Regular use of stimulant drugs can lead to dependence. Other problems include chronic insomnia, impaired memory, personality change, depression, anxiety and psychosis. If the stimulant drug is injected, then the risk of harm increases significantly. Possible consequences include skin infections, HIV, hepatitis, overdose and death.

Stimulant drugs as medications

There are a group of stimulant drugs that are produced as medicines for the treatment of medical disorders such as attention-deficit hyperactivity disorder (ADHD) and narcolepsy. These medications include methylphenidate (brand names include Ritalin® and Concerta®) and dexamfetamine (Adderall® and Dexedrine®). When used as part of medical treatment under clinical supervision, these drugs can be very helpful. Taken without proper supervision, however, they can cause problems similar to illegal stimulant drugs.

Peter's story

Peter is 18 years old, single and living with friends. He works as a manager in a well-known coffee chain and is saving money to go to film school. Peter's friends describe him as shy and Peter regards himself as an introvert. Despite this, Peter has had several successful relationships, although he has been single for 4 months.

Peter doesn't drink alcohol but very occasionally smokes cannabis when out with friends. Last weekend one of his close friends invited him to a house party and mentioned that there would be lots of new people there that he would get on with. With some reluctance he agreed to go and was excited to meet some really interesting people. He was particularly taken by one woman, Kate, and began to flirt with her. After an hour, Kate offered him a line of cocaine. Not wishing to seem 'uncool', Peter accepted, although he had never used cocaine before.

Peter described the next hour as the most extraordinary of his life. After snorting the cocaine he said that 'my brain caught fire' and he suddenly felt as if his mind was working 'ten times as fast' as usual. He felt 'ecstatic' and started talking to three people at the same time, understanding and responding to what each was saying. People seemed fascinated by what he had to say and Kate was 'hanging on every word'. He believed he could feel every nerve ending in his body and that he was 'humming with this incredible energy, like some kind of superhero'.

A little while later, Peter asked Kate for more cocaine but after the second dose, his heart began to 'speed up'. He felt it beating faster and faster until it was 'hammering' in his chest.

He began to panic, thinking that he was having a heart attack, and could feel an intense sharp pain across his chest. Within a few minutes he became 'hysterical' and his friend called an ambulance.

By the time Peter reached the emergency room, he was convinced he was going to die. He was sweating and felt he couldn't breathe. A doctor gave him medication that helped him relax. A few hours later the cocaine had worn off and Peter was left exhausted and embarrassed. As he was no longer a medical risk, the emergency doctor was happy for him to go home after talking to a psychiatrist. As he talked about his experience, he vowed never to use drugs again.

Key messages

- Stimulants are popular and very powerful psychoactive drugs that produce desirable short-term effects for the user.

- Stimulant drugs make the user feel alert, euphoric and full of energy, improve concentration and reduce fatigue.

- Common stimulant drugs include cocaine, amphetamines and ecstasy.

- However, they also cause a range of both short- and long-term harm that can be life-threatening.

- Stimulants are highly addictive and can lead to dependence, withdrawal syndrome and marked tolerance (the need to take larger amounts to achieve the same effect).

Sedatives

Sedative drugs have the opposite effect to stimulants, while still producing powerful psychoactive effects for the user. They make the person feel physically relaxed (slowing their heart rate and lowering blood pressure) and psychologically calm (reducing anxiety), with a sense of serenity and well-being.

Sedative drugs are attractive to people who have feelings that they can't tolerate and want to suppress. By reducing anxiety, sedative drugs can diminish or even temporarily rid the user of difficult thoughts and feelings, making problems seem less overwhelming. They work quickly and can cause a very powerful psychological experience that feels hugely relieving, even if the sedative effect only lasts for a short time.

But sedatives are not only used to take away anxiety and difficult feelings. Some people also enjoy the experience of intoxication that can result when a large quantity of a sedative drug is taken. As the dose is increased, the user becomes disinhibited and their physical coordination is reduced, judgement is impaired and memory becomes unreliable. Sensations such as sounds can be exaggerated and the user can become disorientated and confused. Users may also experience heightened pleasure, a sense of psychological release and enjoyment. For some, being intoxicated is fun, but for others, the loss of control is disturbing and frightening.

Sedative drugs include a wide range of different chemicals that work through different inhibitory receptors in the brain. They have varying strengths, with some causing mild relaxation while others can rapidly lead to unconsciousness. The most commonly used illegal sedating drug across the world, excluding alcohol, is cannabis (see section in this chapter on cannabis). Other groups of sedative drugs, misused for their psychoactive effects, include opioids/opiates, barbiturates, benzodiazepines and 'Z-drugs'. Common sedative drugs and their negative effects are listed in Table 5.2.

Opiate/opioid drugs

Opiate/opioid drugs are powerful sedatives. The term 'opiate' is generally used to describe drugs that have been made from opium derived from poppy plants. Examples include morphine or heroin. By contrast, 'opioid' drugs are entirely synthetically manufactured. Many are used as medications, for example codeine, OxyContin® and tramadol. They have powerful pain-reducing effects and are used for a wide range of medical conditions. They also produce powerful psychoactive effects including sedation and a dream-like emotional state. If prescribed in the correct dose and for the right length of time, opioid-based drugs are safe and extremely helpful medications for pain management.

Opioid/opiate drugs are very dangerous if misused as they can slow or even halt breathing. This is the cause of death in many cases of heroin overdose.

Table 5.2 Common sedative drugs and their associated problems

Drug group	Description	Common names[a]	Short-term problems	Long-term problems
Benzodiazepines	• Synthetic drugs that reduce anxiety and induce sleep • Widely used as medication • Typically available as tablets • Used recreationally for their sedative and disinhibiting effects	Benzos, vallies, roofies, moggies, jellies, blues	Over-sedation, loss of physical coordination, slurred speech, memory loss, disinhibition and risk-taking, accidents, convulsions, coma, overdose and death	Severe dependence if used for long periods, tolerance, withdrawal symptoms
Z-drugs	• Synthetic drugs that work through a similar mechanism to benzodiazepine • Used to treat insomnia • Available as tablets	Zopiclone, zolpiderm	Likely to be similar to benzodiazepines	Little research on risks, but likely to be similar to benzodiazepines
Barbiturates	• Powerful sedatives that work largely through the GABA receptor system • Previously used as medications to treat anxiety, insomnia and epilepsy	Barbs, barbies, sleepers	High risk of overdose because there is only a small difference between the prescribed dose and dose causing over-sedation	As for benzodiazepines, although risks of dependence and overdose are greater
Opiates	• Derived from the opium poppy, opiates are powerful sedatives with strong pain-reducing properties • Heroin is a white or brown powder that can be smoked or dissolved before injecting	Heroin, morphine, gear, smack, junk	Intense 'rush', feeling separated from the world, sedation, slowed breathing and heart rate, overdose and death	Most longer-term harm relates to the way the drug is taken: injecting heroin and other opiates is particularly harmful, increasing the risk of overdose, HIV and hepatitis and spreading infection throughout the body

Drug group	Description	Common names[a]	Short-term problems	Long-term problems
Opioids	• Widely used in medicine for the treatment of pain • Manufactured in tablet, capsule and injectable forms	Usually known by their chemical (e.g. methadone) or brand name	As for opiates	As for opiates
GHB/GBL	• Synthetic chemicals manufactured for use as industrial solvents • Typically available as a liquid that has to be diluted, occasionally available as a powder or paste • Leads to disinhibition, increased libido and sedation • Often sold cheaply as 'shots'	G	There is only a small difference between the dose needed to achieve the desired effects and a dose that results in coma, therefore GHB/GBL users are at high risk of overdose, particularly if they have little experience with the drug	Severe and rapidly developing tolerance and dependence, severe, life-threatening withdrawal symptoms, little research on the long-term effects of use
Anticonvulsants	• Used for the treatment of epilepsy, anxiety and pain • When misused cause disinhibition, euphoria, sedation and relaxation • Produced as capsules and tablets; when misused, sometimes snorted	Usually known by their chemical (e.g. pregabalin, gabapentin) or brand names	Causes sedation, vomiting, insomnia and confusion; risks increase if mixed with other sedatives	Dependence has been reported with pregabalin

a. The terms used for drugs differ over time and from place to place. The examples given were common at the time of writing.
Sources: www.drugscope.org.uk and Royal Society for the Encouragement of Arts, Manufactures and Commerce (2007).

Barbiturates

These drugs are now rarely used because of the risk of overdose and they have been largely replaced in doctors' surgeries by benzodiazepines.

Benzodiazepines

Benzodiazepines are the most commonly prescribed group of sedative drugs and include medications such as diazepam, alprazolam and lorazepam. They work on the inhibitory GABA receptors in the brain to produce a powerful sedative effect. These sedative and anxiety-reducing effects are harnessed in medications that treat anxiety and insomnia.

For people suffering from severe anxiety and distress, for example following bereavement or other crisis, sedative and anxiety-reducing medications can be extremely helpful in relieving symptoms for a short period. Short-term insomnia such as jetlag can also be greatly helped by using a sedative drug with a sleep-inducing effect.

When prescribed for short periods and at the correct dose, these drugs are safe and very useful. They do, however, have the potential to cause severe dependence if taken for too long or at too high a dose. Like the opioid/opiate drugs, if they are misused, they are strong enough to cause life-threatening overdose by stopping a person breathing.

Z-drugs

A similar group of drugs to the benzodiazepines, Z-drugs include zolpidem and zopiclone. The Z-drugs act in the brain in a similar way to benzodiazepines, but are only licensed for the treatment of insomnia. They are thought to have similar risks of dependence as benzodiazepines.

Other sedative drugs

Pregabalin and gabapentin are anticonvulsant drugs used in the treatment of epilepsy. They are also used to treat long-term pain problems, and pregabalin is licensed for the treatment of anxiety. Both drugs produce psychoactive effects and misuse can lead to relaxation, a sense of calm, drowsiness and euphoria. There has been increasing concern about their misuse as they can slow breathing. They can be fatal if taken in large amounts, particularly if mixed with other sedative drugs.

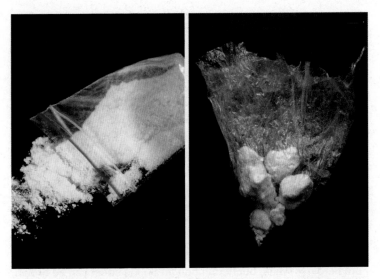

Cocaine is most commonly bought in the form of a white powder (left), which is usually snorted. Crack cocaine is a form of cocaine that can be smoked in a pipe or injected. It is typically sold as crystals, sometimes called 'rocks' (right). It's known as crack because it makes a cracking sound when heated.

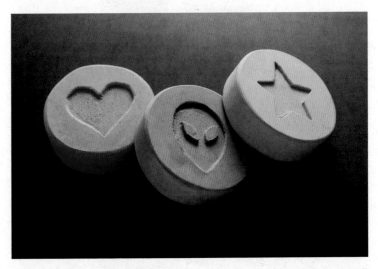

MDMA, also known as ecstasy or molly, is usually sold as small tablets, often printed with designs. It sometimes comes as crystals or powder, which can be white, yellowish or amber.

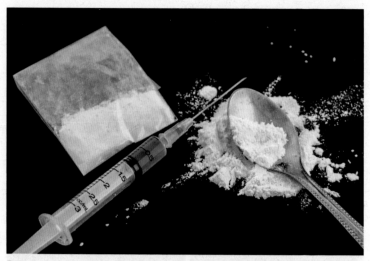

Pure heroin is white, but heroin bought on the street can be brown, black or pinkish-grey. As well as being injected, heroin can also be smoked or snorted.

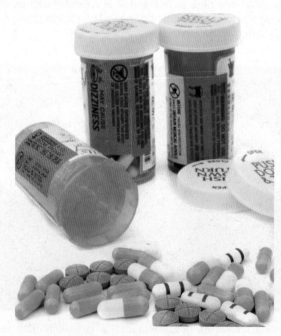

Benzodiazepines are depressant drugs (well-known brand names are Valium®, Xanax® and Klonopin®) that come in tablet or capsule form.

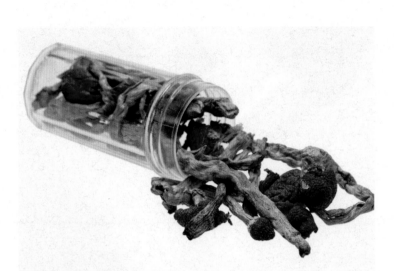

Magic mushrooms, a type of hallucinogen, can be eaten raw or prepared in food or drink.

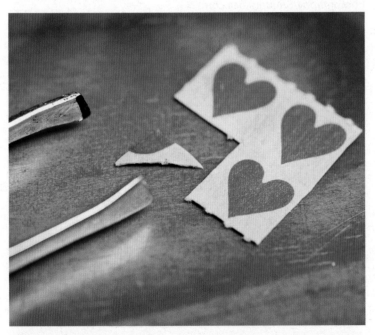

LSD is often added in liquid form to an absorbent surface, such as a small square of blotting paper, which is dissolved on the tongue.

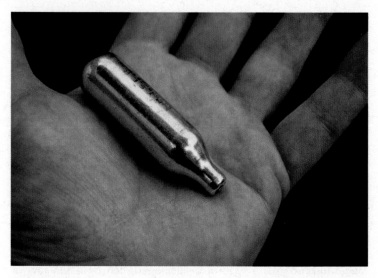

Nitrous oxide, also known as laughing gas, is usually sold in small silver canisters and inhaled using a balloon (image from Lenscap Photography/Shutterstock.com).

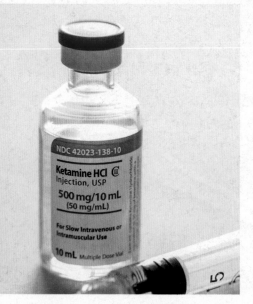

Ketamine can be obtained in the form of a white powder or as a clear, odourless liquid.

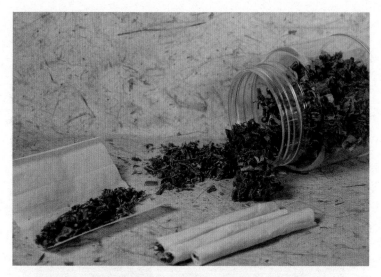

Natural cannabis prepared for smoking. Cigarette papers are used to roll joints.

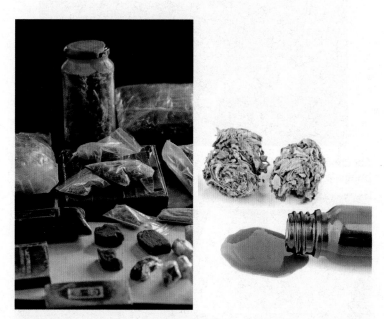

Cannabis can come in a variety of forms, including leaf, resin (left) and oil (right).

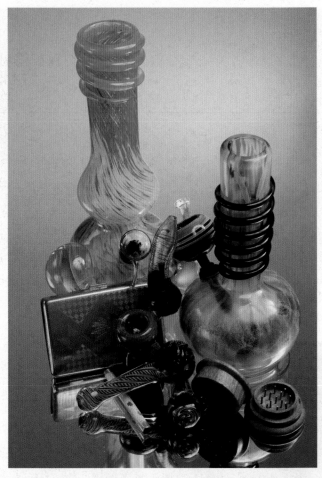

Cannabis can be smoked using a range of paraphernalia, including bongs, pipes (above) and cigarette papers (below).

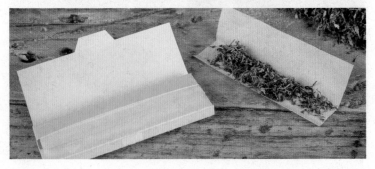

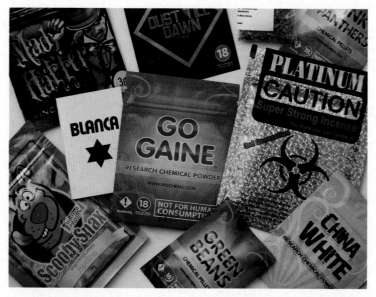

The bright packaging of the so-called 'legal highs' is similar to that used to market alcopops.

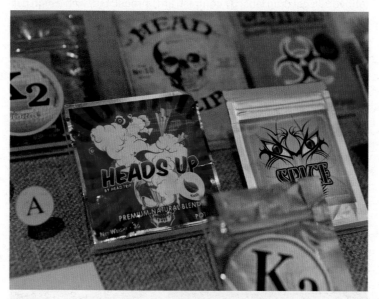

Synthetic cannabis comes in various strengths, and can be much stronger than natural cannabis.

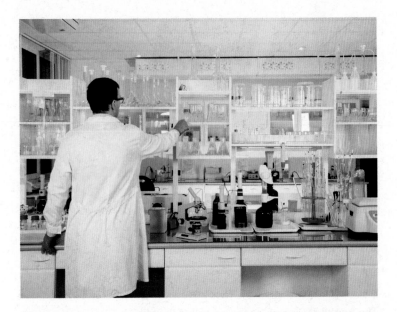

Pharmaceutical medications are manufactured in laboratories with strict rules regarding hygiene and cleanliness to avoid contamination (above). Illegal drug labs, by contrast, are unregulated, with a high risk of accidental contamination (below).

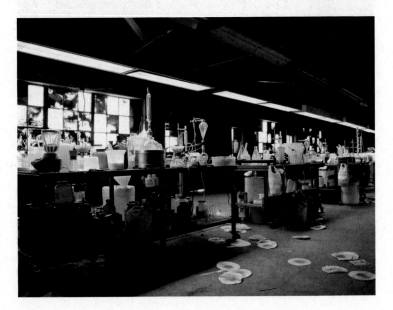

How are sedative drugs used?

Sedative drugs can be used in a variety of ways. Heroin can be snorted, smoked and injected (see the colour section). Many of the opioids can also be taken by these routes, although sedatives such as the benzodiazepines tend to be taken as tablets.

Users sometimes mix sedative drugs with stimulant drugs, in a way that reduces the unwanted effects of the drugs. By mixing crack cocaine and heroin in the same syringe for injection, a practice known as 'speedballing', the user is trying to get a better experience. The sedating heroin reduces the unwanted agitation caused by the stimulating crack cocaine. There are many examples of drug users combining drugs with different effects to improve their using experience. However, combining different drugs usually increases the risk of harm as different chemicals mix together in unpredictable ways.

What problems can sedative drugs cause?

Immediate and short-term problems

Sedative drugs are very dangerous if taken in large amounts or mixed with other sedatives. They can dramatically slow breathing and make users feel very sleepy and over-sedated. Overdose can be fatal, as breathing can stop altogether. The risk of overdose is particularly high if two or more sedatives are taken at the same time; for example, a benzodiazepine with alcohol.

For people who are dependent on a sedative drug, severe withdrawal effects can occur if the drug is stopped too quickly. This can be very dangerous, particularly for benzodiazepines and barbiturates, where rapid withdrawal can lead to seizures.

Problems from repeated use

Sedative drugs like heroin can cause severe dependence, with marked tolerance (the need to take larger and larger amounts to achieve a similar effect). Repeated use of sedative drugs can lead to depression and, paradoxically, increase anxiety over time.

Some of the harm from repeated use depends on the way the drug is taken. Injecting is particularly dangerous, risking skin infections, blood poisoning, HIV and hepatitis.

Jill's story

Jill is 20 years old and working in her first job since leaving university. She was thrilled when she found a job in advertising, something she had always hoped to do.

For as long as Jill can remember, she has experienced anxiety. Even as a small child she remembers being easily frightened and becoming distraught when things did not go her way. Her mother had always been 'totally stressed' and Jill assumed that 'nerves run in my family'. During her first school exams, Jill experienced a panic attack and described this as 'like dying'. She sought help and completed a course of cognitive–behavioural therapy, which allowed her to manage her anxiety most of the time.

Despite her anxiety about examinations, Jill did well academically and went to her university of choice. Unfortunately, her first year was 'a total nightmare' because her anxiety returned in the new setting and interfered with making friends and studying. Jill felt 'socially crippled' and thought about starting more psychological work. Instead, another student, who also had problems with anxiety, gave Jill a 5 mg tablet of diazepam (often known by the brand name Valium®). For Jill, the diazepam worked 'like magic' and, for the first time she could remember, she felt entirely free of anxiety. After this experience, Jill went to her GP for a 2-week supply of diazepam. She used the tablets for social events and also before tutorials to keep her anxiety at bay. Her GP prescribed one further week of diazepam but explained that it would be the last prescription because of the risk of addiction. He suggested that Jill should try psychological treatment again and she knew this was the right advice.

However, she was so busy with her studies that she could not see how she could find the time to attend therapy. Besides, the diazepam worked so well that she thought that as long as she was careful and used the tablets sparingly, she could manage without problems. Jill bought diazepam from the internet, and for the next few months everything went well. Around this time Jill first mixed diazepam with alcohol. She found this gave her a very pleasant feeling of being intoxicated, relaxed and carefree. 'It was just a lovely, dreamy feeling, I'd never had that before', she said. Socialising was easy and she started a relationship with her very first boyfriend.

In retrospect, Jill admits she knew her diazepam use was getting out of control. She began to use more frequently, typically using the excuse that things were particularly stressful for her that day. She also used bigger doses, convincing herself that the internet-bought diazepam was not as strong as that previously prescribed by the GP.

By the time Jill started work, she was using 50–70 mg of diazepam each day – much larger doses than would usually be prescribed. She was taking two or three tablets each morning just to keep her anxiety at a tolerable level, and was on the verge of resigning from her job because the thought of going to work was overwhelming. Jill was also drinking far too much alcohol.

Realising that her diazepam use was out of control, Jill agreed to start treatment and let the clinic contact her GP and employers to negotiate time off work. She turned to the psychological approaches that had worked for her in her teens and completed a detoxification programme for both alcohol and diazepam.

Jill still experiences some anxiety, but can generally manage it using psychological techniques. After 7 weeks away from work, Jill is now on a graded return, apprehensive but excited about getting on with life.

Key messages

- Sedative drugs make the user feel calm, relaxed and serene. At higher doses, the user can feel disinhibited and lose physical coordination.

- Sedative drugs can be attractive for people who experience anxiety or have difficult thoughts or feelings they want to suppress.

- Common sedative drugs include cannabis, opiate/opioids (e.g. heroin) and benzodiazepines (e.g. Valium®).

- Because they slow breathing, sedatives are very dangerous in overdose, particularly if they are mixed with other sedatives.

- Repeated use of sedative drugs can lead to severe dependence.

Cannabis

Cannabis is a sedative drug but, because of its popularity, particularly in adolescence, it warrants its own section.

What is cannabis?

Cannabis is a sedative drug produced from flowering plants grown across the globe, both naturally and in specially devised settings, such as industrial greenhouses. Cannabis is the most commonly used psychoactive drug in the world (excluding the legal drugs alcohol, caffeine and nicotine). The United Nations estimates that nearly 180 million people used cannabis in the past year, far more than amphetamines (34 million), opioids (33 million) and ecstasy (17 million) (United Nations Office on Drugs and Crime, 2014).

The main psychoactive agent in cannabis is tetrahydro-cannabinol (THC), although there are other psychoactive constituents. Cannabis works directly on cannabinoid receptors in the brain to produce a range of short-term desired effects, including relaxation, disinhibition, uncontrollable laughter, altered perception of time (usually slowed), introspection and (occasionally) hallucinations.

Different types of cannabis

The cannabis plant has a large number of varieties, each with different strengths. The term 'skunk' is used to describe a particularly strong-smelling variety. Skunk cannabis can have three to four times more THC than ordinary cannabis. This higher THC content gives skunk greater psychoactive effects but also the potential for greater harm. For example, there is emerging evidence of a link between skunk and mental illness. Research suggests that the risk of psychotic breakdown is three times higher in people who smoke skunk cannabis, compared with people who don't Di Forti *et al*, 2015). The risk increases further if skunk is smoked every day. Common types of cannabis and their consequences for the user are displayed in Table 5.3.

How is cannabis used?

Cannabis is produced in three main forms, directly from the leaves (known as weed or pot), as a resin (known as hash) or as an oil. It is most commonly consumed by smoking it in a rolled cigarette (called a 'joint') with or without tobacco, but can also be smoked in a pipe or bong (glass water pipe) or prepared in food or drinks. See the colour section for more photos of cannabis and items associated with it.

Cannabis as a medicine

Natural cannabis has been shown to have potential medical use, particularly in treating nausea, stimulating appetite,

Table 5.3 Common types of cannabis

Drug	Description	Common names[a]	Short-term problems	Long-term problems
Cannabis (natural)	• Produced from a naturally occuring psychoactive plant as leaves, flower buds, resin or oil • Typically smoked or eaten • Effects include relaxation, disinhibition, perceptual changes, introspection and (occasionally) hallucinations • Cannabis-based medications treat nausea, stimulate appetite, alleviate muscle spasms in multiple sclerosis and reduce long-term pain	• Leaves and buds are called weed, marijuana, pot, ganja or grass • Resin is usually called hash or hashish • Stronger varieties are often termed 'skunk' and command higher prices	• Sedation, nausea, palpitations, dizziness, bloodshot eyes, low blood pressure, hunger ('the munchies'), anxiety, panic, confusion, paranoia, insomnia and (rarely) psychosis • Short-term problems vary according to the level of THC content	• Tolerance and dependence • Withdrawal symptoms tend to be psychological rather than physical and not life-threatening • Heavy, long-term use can result in loss of motivation, poor concentration and memory problems • Increases risk of psychosis in people who already have mental health problems • Might increase the risk of developing psychotic illness in vulnerable individuals • Long-term problems relate to level of THC content
Synthetic cannabinoids	• Non-psychoactive plant material sprayed with chemicals that work at the same brain receptors as natural cannabis • Has various strengths, can be much stronger than natural cannabis	• Known by a wide variety of brand names (e.g. Spice, K2, Black Mamba)	• As for natural cannabis, although emerging evidence suggests it's more likely to result in problems including psychosis	• Little evidence available at present • Lkely to be similar to natural cannabis but may cause greater mental health problems

a. The terms used for drugs differ over time and from place to place. The examples given were common at the time of writing.
Sources: www.drugscope.org.uk and Royal Society for the Encouragement of Arts, Manufactures and Commerce (2007).

reducing long-term pain and alleviating muscle spasms in multiple sclerosis (Borgelt *et al*, 2013). Medical cannabis is usually available as a tablet or spray and is licensed in several countries, including the UK and parts of the USA.

Synthetic cannabis

The past decade has seen the marketing of huge numbers of synthetic cannabinoid products. These drugs chemically mimic the effects of natural cannabis. With brand names like Spice and Black Mamba or simply labelled as herbal incense, synthetic cannabinoids contain no actual cannabis plant or THC. Instead, they are produced by spraying everyday plant material with psychoactive chemicals that work on the same brain receptors as THC. Synthetic cannabinoids can be smoked in a cigarette or bong just like traditional natural cannabis.

Many different chemicals of varying strengths have been detected in synthetic cannabinoid products, leading to a very unpredictable user experience. There are concerns that synthetic cannabinoid products might be more harmful than traditional natural cannabis. Hallucinations and psychosis (losing touch with reality) in particular seem to be more common with synthetic cannabinoids. As they are relatively new to the drug market, there has been very little research on their safety.

What problems can cannabis and synthetic cannabis cause?

Immediate and short-term problems

Unwanted short-term effects include nausea, dizziness, sedation, low blood pressure, palpitations, bloodshot eyes, hunger ('the munchies'), anxiety, panic, paranoia, insomnia and (rarely) psychosis. There is emerging evidence that synthetic cannabinoids cause more severe problems, including agitation, psychosis and heart problems (Harris & Brown, 2013).

Problems with repeated use

Heavy, repeated use of cannabis can lead to reduced motivation, poor concentration and memory problems. There is some controversy regarding a link with major mental illnesses such as schizophrenia, but repeated cannabis use does increase the risk of psychosis in some people (Manrique-Garcia *et al*, 2012).

There is currently very little information on the effects of repeated use of synthetic cannabinoids, but the risks seem to be higher than for natural cannabis (Winstock & Barratt, 2013).

Amelia's story

Amelia is 16 years old and sitting school examinations in 6 months. She has been brought to the clinic by her parents, who are very worried about her. Previously, Amelia was the 'perfect daughter', doing well academically and with friends her parents liked. Her parents explained that Amelia 'fell in with a druggy crowd' a year ago and that, since then, things have gone downhill. They describe her as verbally aggressive, irritable and secretive, and were upset when she pierced her nose and had a small infinity sign tattooed on her shoulder.

While her parents talked, Amelia sat motionless, scowling at the floor. She made no attempt to join in the conversation, but looked furious. Her parents agreed to wait outside while I talked to Amelia on her own. The moment her parents left the room, Amelia sighed deeply and made eye contact for the first time. I asked if she was happy to talk and she looked at me intensely, deciding whether to bother. Fortunately, her anger had left the room along with her parents and with the slightest nod of agreement, Amelia started to tell me about herself.

She admitted that she had become bored with her school friends and had met people from another school. She had sought out 'people who think for themselves' and, after starting a relationship with a boy who smoked a lot of cannabis, started smoking herself. Amelia 'loved' the feeling of being 'stoned' and her use had rapidly increased. Some of her school friends thought she was 'cool' for smoking, while others had stayed away, telling her she was 'a loser'.

Amelia did not think her cannabis use was an issue and felt it helped her relax. She admitted that she was now smoking most days and felt 'a bit twitchy' if she went for more than a few days without a joint. Her boyfriend bought all the cannabis for her. Amelia explained that she did not want to make any changes to her drug use and did not want to see me or anyone from my team.

I wasn't sure if I would see Amelia again, but a few months later she returned without her parents. Since we last met, her cannabis use had 'gone out of control' and she had begun experiencing 'weird thoughts'. She felt that strangers were staring at her in the street and whispering to each other that she was 'a bitch'. Amelia knew that cannabis could cause paranoia but didn't want to cut back, as she thought her boyfriend would like her less. As the thoughts intensified, she told her boyfriend about them, but he told her not to worry.

Ten days before we met for the second time, her boyfriend ended the relationship, saying that he had met someone else. Amelia did not feel particularly upset as she was getting fed up with 'just sitting around and smoking', but her supply of cannabis abruptly ended. Her last joint had been 10 days ago and she had been feeling anxious, agitated and unable to sleep. In desperation, she went online and bought synthetic cannabis that made her feel 'messed up': panicky, paranoid and frightened. While stoned on the synthetic cannabis, she thought zombies were trying to break into her room and believed she could hear them scratching on her bedroom walls at night.

Amelia agreed to meet me again and, although not agreeing to stop using cannabis altogether, wanted to talk about cutting down. Unfortunately, Amelia did not come to her next appointment and left a message saying that she was back with her boyfriend and did not want treatment after all. I wrote to Amelia and left a message on her phone, but did not hear back. Her parents have been in touch and feel that overall she is doing better, but have asked for an appointment to discuss how they can encourage Amelia back into treatment.

I'm hopeful that Amelia will come back to treatment, although in the end it is up to her. In the meantime, I continue to support her parents.

Key messages

- Cannabis is the world's most commonly used illegal drug and is made from the leaves and buds of the cannabis plant.

- Cannabis is usually smoked and the user experiences relaxation, introspection, changes in the perception of time, uncontrollable laughter and (occasionally) hallucinations.

- The main psychoactive chemical in cannabis is called tetrahydrocannabinol (THC). Some types of cannabis have much higher quantities of THC and these are often called skunk.

- Cannabis-related harm such as paranoia and psychosis is more likely with higher THC content. Long-term heavy use leads to a loss of motivation and memory problems.

- Synthetic cannabinoid drugs are also available. Generally stronger than traditional natural cannabis, they might also be more harmful.

Hallucinogens

What are hallucinogenic drugs?

Hallucinogenic drugs produce two important types of perceptual experiences: distortions and hallucinations. As well as accompanying hallucinogenic drug use, they can also occur in physical and mental illnesses, including schizophrenia, severe sleep deprivation and (less commonly) as a side-effect of certain medications.

Distortions happen when the brain misinterprets information from the senses and can apply to anything we see, touch, hear, taste or smell. Colours can become more intense, patterns more complex, objects can change size or shape, and noises can be amplified and distorted. The senses detect something but the brain gets mixed up trying to understand it. Distortions can be pleasant and intriguing, or distressing, unsettling and frightening.

Hallucinations occur when the brain sees, hears or feels something that is not really there. Unlike distortions, there is no misinterpretation. Instead, the brain makes up the sensation. Hallucinations, like distortions, can also happen in all five senses, although psychoactive drugs are more likely to cause auditory and visual hallucinations. Hallucinations can be subtle and amusing or overwhelming and terrifying.

Hallucinogenic drugs can sometimes confuse the brain so much that it mixes up different senses. The technical term is synaesthesia and the brain becomes so confused that people 'hear' colours or 'see' sounds.

Users often describe intoxication using hallucinogens as a 'trip', to indicate a journey away from reality. If the hallucinations and distortions become too intense or frightening, users might call this a 'bad trip'. Hallucinogen users often describe deeply reflective, emotionally insightful or spiritual experiences when using and this can be a powerful attraction of these drugs.

Types of hallucinogens

The best-known hallucinogenic drug is lysergic acid diethylamide, often called LSD or acid. LSD was first synthesised in 1938, with the hope that it could be a useful medicine. Once the powerful hallucinogenic effects were discovered, however, it became a popular recreational drug, strongly associated with the counter-culture movement of the 1960s. Some used the powerful effects of LSD to develop and enhance creativity. Aldous Huxley, Robert Graves and, perhaps most famously, Timothy Leary were vocal advocates of the drug's potential to enhance personal growth. Other hallucinogens include so-called 'magic mushrooms', which contain the drug psilocybin, and the cactus peyote. Common hallucinogens and their consequences are listed in Table 5.4.

In the early 1990s, American pharmacologist Alexander Shulgin and his wife Ann Shulgin wrote a book titled *PIHKAL: A Chemical Love Story*. *PIHKAL* was effectively a cookbook for psychoactive drugs, containing hundreds of recipes explaining in detail the chemical processes to manufacture different drugs. Alexander Shulgin, sometimes credited with introducing ecstasy to the USA, was particularly interested in hallucinogens and took many of the drugs he synthesised himself. Over his career he synthesised over 200 different compounds and his work paved the way for both researchers and those interested in recreational drug use.

Since then, numerous other hallucinogenic drugs have appeared on the market. Some of these newer drugs are extremely powerful, with even very small doses producing prolonged hallucinogenic effects. They can induce overwhelming and frightening perceptual disturbances lasting hours or even days.

The brain mechanisms underpinning hallucinogenic drugs are poorly understood but are thought to involve the serotonin neurotransmitter system.

How are hallucinogens used?

LSD causes psychoactive effects in low doses of 50–150 micrograms (rather than milligrams or even grams for most other psychoactive drugs). It is usually produced by placing a small drop of the chemical on a small square of blotting paper or on a sugar cube (see the colour section for an example). This dries and can later be consumed by dissolving on the tongue. Once taken, LSD takes about half an hour to work but the effects can last several hours.

Magic mushrooms (see the colour section) can be consumed by eating them or preparing them in a drink. Every year there are fatal poisonings due to inexperienced mushroom pickers eating poisonous mushrooms they mistakenly thought were the hallucinogenic type.

The newer synthetic hallucinogens are produced as tablets, powders or on blotting paper, often with brand names or labelled as research chemicals.

What problems can hallucinogens cause?

Immediate and short-term problems

Taking hallucinogens can lead to what users refer to as a bad trip. Distortions and hallucinations become intense to the point of being terrifying. Users can experience extreme agitation and psychosis as they lose touch with reality. Occasionally, accidental death results directly from hallucinogen ingestion when a user, either in a state of intoxication or fleeing from an imaginary threat, fatally injures themselves, for example by falling from a height.

Users sometimes relate having a bad trip with their emotional state immediately before taking the drug and some users go to great length to use hallucinogens in a carefully created, calm environment, perhaps choosing particular music to listen to. The newer, and generally stronger, hallucinogens seem more likely to cause problems, including nausea, vomiting, severe agitation and psychosis.

Problems with repeated use

Heavy, repeated use of hallucinogens can cause longer-term problems. Some users describe 'flashbacks' weeks, months or even years after they last used hallucinogens. During these flashbacks, the user re-experiences some of the distortions and hallucinations without having taken any drug. Users generally find these flashbacks disturbing, although they usually become less intense and less frequent over time.

Hallucinogen persisting perceptual disorder (HPPD) is even more severe than a flashback. With HPPD, the trip just doesn't stop. Users experience constant distortions and hallucinations, including bright auras around objects, flashing lights or light 'trails' that continue without a break for weeks or months after the drug use. Symptoms can range from mildly annoying to overwhelming and distressing. HPPD remains a controversial

Table 5.4 Common hallucinogenic drugs and their associated problems

Drug	Description	Common names[a]	Short-term problems	Long-term problems
LSD	• Synthetic drug • Usually applied to small pieces of blotting paper, also available as a liquid or pellets • Effects include altered mood, perceptual distortions and hallucinations that can last for hours	Acid, trips, tabs, microdots	Effects can be intense and frightening, a 'bad trip' can result in disturbing imagery, persecutory thinking and extreme anxiety, intoxicated users can accidentally or deliberately injure themselves, tolerance develops quickly	Persisting or returning distortions and hallucinations, concentration and memory problems, people with existing mental health problems may be susceptible to harm, no evidence of dependence or withdrawal symptoms
Psilocybin (magic mushrooms)	• Usually harvested from the wild • Main types are 'liberty cap' and the more potent 'fly agaric' • Liberty cap can be eaten raw, cooked in food or made into tea • Produces efects similar to (but usually less intense than) LSD	Liberties, shrooms, liberty cap, philosopher's stone	Nausea, bad trip (see LSD), fly agaric ingestion can be fatal, accidental poisoning from eating other mushrooms by mistake, injury while intoxicated	No evidence of dependence or withdrawal symptoms, people with existing mental health problems may be particularly susceptible to harm
Salvia divinorum	• Plant from Central America that can be chewed, smoked or prepared as a drink • Effects include perceptual distortions and hallucinations	Herbal ecstasy, herbal high, holy sage	Headache, nausea, injury while intoxicated, agitation, panic (particularly related to frightening hallucinations)	Little research, no current evidence of dependence, people with existing mental health problems might be particularly susceptible to harm
New hallucinogenic drugs	• Large number of new drugs that cause effects similar to and sometimes stronger than LSD	2CB, 2CI, DMT, DXM, research chemicals	As for LSD, but may be more intense and last longer	As for LSD, but may be more intense and last longer

a. The terms used for drugs differ over time and from place to place. The examples given were common at the time of writing.
Sources: given: www.drugscope.org.uk and Royal Society for the Encouragement of Arts, Manufactures and Commerce (2007).

diagnosis, with some clinicians believing it is more related to underlying anxiety. Only a small number of hallucinogen users seem to be affected in this way, but the experience for those few can be debilitating.

Some researchers suggest that heavy use of hallucinogens can cause other brain problems, such as memory difficulties. There is no evidence that hallucinogens cause the dependence or withdrawal syndromes seen with many other drugs. Most of what we know about hallucinogens is based on traditional drugs such as LSD and psilocybin. We know very little about the newer synthetic hallucinogens, although they seem to be more powerful and potentially more harmful.

Rajiv's story

Rajiv is a 19-year-old man who came to see me after his best friend begged him to get help. He arrives on time, casually dressed in a hoodie, jeans and trainers, looking tired but keen to help me understand his situation.

He begins by saying that he really enjoys using hallucinogens, which he has used most weeks for the past 2 years. He never drinks alcohol or uses other drugs and takes care of his health by consuming a large number of vitamins and mineral pills he buys from a health food store.

For Rajiv, hallucinogenic drugs are unlike other drugs because they reveal the 'inner workings', put him in a 'spiritual state' and give him 'a different perspective on the universe'.

Rajiv talks with enthusiasm about his hallucinogen experiences. Objects grow and shrink or emit bright colours and 'melt round the edges'. Colours and sounds become exceptionally vivid. Patterns, such as those on wallpaper and curtains, gently move 'like the sea', changing shape to form cartoon-like geometrical patterns. Light trails burst from his hands 'like sparklers' when he moves them and he feels deeply meditative. He greatly enjoys these experiences.

If he takes strong hallucinogens, Rajiv experiences bizarre, complex hallucinations. He sometimes sees 'ghosts' of people he used to know or even 'fantastical visions' including detailed historical or futuristic scenes. Sometimes he can become directly involved but mostly he watches 'like the best cinema ever'. He finds these experiences 'mind-blowing' but admits they are occasionally too intense, sinister and even frightening.

Rajiv denies that he has any problems using hallucinogens and plans to continue using them. He likes to think of himself as a 'psychonaut' exploring the 'final frontier of consciousness'. His friends, however, have a different view.

Rajiv's best friend doesn't use drugs and is worried that Rajiv has 'messed up his head' and is becoming a 'space cadet'. He thinks his personality has changed as a result of his drug use and is frustrated that Rajiv does not realise what is happening to him.

We finish the assessment with Rajiv telling me about all the different types of hallucinogens he has taken as well as the ones he hopes to take in the future. He listens respectfully as I talk him through the risks, but says he does not need any help and knows what he is doing. Like many 'psychonauts', Rajiv has a very detailed knowledge of hallucinogens and their chemistry and is only too happy to talk about them. Rajiv offers to visit me now and again to keep me up to date.

Just keeping a conversation going with Rajiv might be the best I can do for the moment and he is pleased when I agree to see him again in a few weeks.

Key messages

- Hallucinogens are powerful psychoactive drugs that make the brain misinterpret sensations (distortions) or experience sensations when there is nothing there (hallucinations).
- They can cause confusion, disorientation and a loss of touch with reality.
- Experiences can be very intense and frightening (a bad trip).
- Hallucinogens don't cause dependence but can damage the brain if used repeatedly.
- Accidental injury while intoxicated is probably the greatest risk.

Dissociatives

What are dissociative drugs?

Dissociative drugs, like hallucinogens, cause confusion, changes in sensations, trance-like feelings and even out-of-body or near-death experiences. Unlike hallucinogens, however, they do not typically cause hallucinations.

Dissociation is a term used to describe an experience in which mental processes are separated, resulting in one group of mental processes functioning independently from the others. There are only a few commonly used dissociative drugs, including ketamine and nitrous oxide (Table 5.5). Other, less common dissociative drugs include phencyclidine (PCP) and methoxetamine. These drugs cause similar effects but are rarely seen in current drug markets.

Ketamine

Ketamine was developed in 1962 as an anaesthetic. It was initially popular because it did not slow breathing and the effects only lasted a short time – perfect for quick operations. It fell out of favour because on waking from their operation, patients often described vivid nightmares. It is still used in certain medical settings such as emergency rooms and in battlefield medicine, and is common in veterinary medicine.

When ketamine is used illicitly for its psychoactive effect, users describe a range of effects including a floaty, relaxed feeling and intense sounds and colours. At higher doses, the anaesthetic effects of ketamine take over and users are sometimes paralysed, unable to move or feel their bodies.

Many users describe an intense psychological experience called the 'K hole' during which they feel as though they're floating outside their body and experience intense distortions and disorientation. Many ketamine users consider the K hole a rewarding and even spiritual psychological state and will adjust their dose to reach it. For others, the K hole can be very distressing, with some users feeling that they are dying or have already died and are seeing the world from the afterlife. As with most drugs, repeated use leads to tolerance and regular ketamine users find it increasingly difficult to attain the K hole experience.

Nitrous oxide and other inhalants

Inhalants are a group of drugs that are almost exclusively used by breathing them in or sniffing them directly from a container. They include solvents, aerosols and gases. Inhalants appeal to younger users because they are cheap and easy to get hold of. Different drugs appeal to different ages. Glue, lighter fluid and aerosol cans are most common in 12- to 15-year-olds, nitrous oxide is most common in 16- to 17-year-olds and amyl nitirite ('poppers') is mainly used by adults.

Table 5.5 Common dissociative drugs and their associated problems

Drug	What is it?	Common names[a]	Short-term problems	Long-term problems
Ketamine	• Synthetic drug widely used in medicine and vetinary settings • Misused as a powder or more rarely tablet or liquid, can be injected • Intense dissociative effects, moderate euphoria, sedation and reduced pain • Effects last around 30min	Ket, K, Special K	Confusion, agitation, nausea, accidental injury due to inability to feel pain, over-sedation, inability to move, intoxication can be very frightening (users can feel they are dying or have died), risks increase if mixed with sedative drugs	Bladder damage causing frequent, painful urination, severe abdominal pains ('K cramps'), some evidence of memory and concentration problems and psychological dependence, unclear if physical withdrawal symptoms occur
Nitrous oxide	• Colourless gas used as dental anaesthetic and in aerosols • Usually inhaled from a balloon filled from canisters (whippets) • Very short-acting: light-headedness, relaxation and euphoria, loss of coordination	Nitrous, hippy crack, nos	Nausea, dizziness, collapse, accidental injury following collapse, risk of death if used directly from canister (nitrous oxide displaces oxygen from the lungs), risks increase if mixed with sedative drugs	Vitamin B12 deficiency that, in severe cases, can lead to nerve damage
Other inhalants	• Range of substances that are sniffed or breathed in • Volatile solvents (e.g. paint thinners, cleaning fluids, glue, lighter fluid), aerosol propellants, butane, amyl nitrite	Usually known by brand name of product; amyl nitrite is referred to as poppers	Nausea, vomiting, severe headaches, convulsions, occasional death from throat spasm, suffocation or acute heart problems	Damage to skin around nose and mouth, damage to organs including liver, kidney and brain, (occasionally) tolerance and dependence

a. The terms used for drugs differ over time and from place to place. The examples given were common at the time of writing. Sources: www.drugscope.org.uk and Royal Society for the Encouragement of Arts, Manufactures and Commerce (2007).

The effects of intoxication are brief, usually only lasting a few minutes. Dizziness, loss of coordination, slurred speech, euphoria, disinhibition and confusion are common. Because the effects only last a short time, users often take many doses over a few hours.

Nitrous oxide is one of the most popular inhalants. Known as laughing gas, it is a colourless, slightly sweet-smelling drug used in dental surgeries and in whipped cream canisters. Laughing gas parties were popular from the 19th century onwards and nitrous oxide has recently revived in popularity in the UK. Inhaling it makes the users feel briefly light-headed, relaxed, disinhibited, giggly, physically uncoordinated and euphoric. It is unclear how it works in the brain, as it affects many different neurotransmitters.

How are dissociatives used?

Ketamine is usually sold as a powder and snorted, although it is rarely, and dangerously, injected. Only a small amount is needed for the desired effect and users talk of taking a 'bump' of ketamine, rather than a 'line' as you would hear about for cocaine.

Inhalants can be taken in a number of ways, including sniffing the substance from a container, breathing it directly into the mouth or nose, or inhaling it from a balloon or plastic bag. Nitrous oxide is usually inhaled from a pre-filled balloon. Occasionally, people inhale directly from the canister using a mask. This is extremely dangerous, as it can rapidly starve the brain of oxygen as the nitrous oxide displaces air from the lungs. This can lead to death.

What problems do dissociative drugs cause?

Problems with immediate and short-term use

Dissociative drugs such as ketamine cause sedation, problems with coordination and reduced feelings of pain. Accidental harm and even death can result because users hurt themselves without noticing. Deaths by drowning and from falls have been reported.

The short-term problems associated with inhalants include severe headache, nausea, vomiting and convulsions. Occasionally, inhaling solvents can cause a spasm of the throat, leading to suffocation. Nitrous oxide impairs physical coordination, and injury from falling over while intoxicated is one of the main risks of the drug. Using nitrous oxide in an enclosed space or inhaling it directly from the cylinder can lead to unconsciousness or death.

The risks from dissociative drugs are increased if they are mixed with sedating drugs such as alcohol or benzodiazepines.

Problems with repeated use

Ketamine is linked to bladder damage (see Greg's story on pp. 75–76). Although the mechanisms are unclear, heavy users describe pain on urination, a need to urinate more often (up to four or five times an hour) and blood-stained urine. These symptoms develop over time and are caused by severe damage to the bladder lining. Occasionally, the bladder becomes damaged beyond repair and reconstructive surgery is needed. Another problem seen in heavy ketamine users is brief but severe abdominal pain, often known to users as 'K cramps'. It is not yet known why they happen.

Both bladder damage and K cramps are extremely painful and distressing, but ketamine itself is an anaesthetic and, like all anaesthetics, it reduces pain. Users can find themselves in a desperate, inescapable trap. Although ketamine is damaging their bodies and causing severe pain, it also brings brief relief from that pain. The user can end up chasing their tail as they take more and more ketamine to control their pain, while at the same time causing further bladder damage. Ketamine users sometimes present to the clinic using huge amounts of ketamine, without which they are in agony. It usually takes the prescription of a different painkiller and referral to a urologist to sort things out. It is not yet clear whether ketamine causes physical dependence, but users report psychological dependence. Depression, anxiety and memory problems have also been described.

Regular use of inhalants can damage the liver and kidneys, as well as the skin around the nose and mouth. Tolerance and dependence have been occasionally reported. Heavy, regular use of nitrous oxide can cause memory problems and can also lead to vitamin B12 deficiency, which itself can cause nerve damage.

Anita's story

Anita is 14 years old and lives with her parents and older brother, Sanjay. She attends her local school, which she enjoys, and has plenty of friends. Recently, Anita has begun to notice boys and they have begun to notice her. She is now invited to lots of parties but her parents only allow her to go occasionally, and then only with her best friend Deepti, who they have known since she was a baby and trust to be a good influence.

Last Saturday, Anita and Deepti went to a friend's birthday party. The party was at their friend's house and the parents were there to supervise and enforce a strict 'no alcohol' rule. Despite this, a few of the boys brought bottles of vodka hidden in their jackets to add to their drinks. Both girls had a great time and later that evening were invited upstairs by some of the 'cool' boys to smoke cigarettes. They climbed out of one of the bedroom windows onto a flat roof to chat and flirt.

One of the boys asked Anita and Deepti if they wanted to try some 'nos'. Not wishing to seem boring, the girls agreed without really understanding what he meant. One of the boys filled a balloon from a small canister and inhaled the contents. Within seconds, he began giggling and stumbling. Everyone tried one balloon. Anita didn't really enjoy the effects. It gave her a headache and she decided it was time for her to go home. Deepti was keen to stay and spend more time with the boys and persuaded Anita to stay a little longer. Several balloons later, one of the boys tried to show off by standing on one leg, but slipped and fell from the roof. Everyone panicked and started screaming. Fortunately, the boy only fell one floor and landed in a bush, but he broke his arm. An ambulance was called and the horrified parents sent everyone home.

The next day, Anita felt 'strange in my head' and was very shaken by the previous night. She was shocked how easily she had accepted nitrous oxide and that she had believed the boys when they said 'it's not even a drug'. She told her parents everything. To her surprise, they listened carefully, making helpful suggestions as to how Anita could stand up for herself and make better choices. Antia has decided not to use nitrous oxide or other drugs again.

Deepti felt differently. She was excited to tell her classmates about the party and what had happened. She did not dare tell her parents because they would stop her from going out. Instead, Deepti planned to meet the boys secretly, excited by how cool and grown up they seemed.

Key messages

- Dissociative drugs cause disorientation, perceptual disturbances, trance-like feelings and even out-of-body or near-death experiences, but rarely hallucinations.

- Nitrous oxide and ketamine are the most commonly misused dissociative drugs.

- Intoxication causes confusion and a loss of physical coordination, which can lead to accidental injury.

- Long-term ketamine use can damage the bladder.

- Long-term nitrous oxide use can cause memory problems and vitamin deficiency.

Rise of the synthetics

Legal highs, club drugs, research chemicals and novel psychoactive substances

The past 40 years has seen the manufacture of a large number of synthetic drugs intended for recreational use. Labelled variously designer drugs, legal highs, club drugs, research chemicals and novel psychoactive substances, they have two things in common. First, they attempt to mimic the effects of 'traditional' drugs, such as cocaine and cannabis. Second, they are produced specifically for recreational purposes, with no intention on the part of the manufacturers to give any medical benefits. They are, essentially, drugs for fun.

Some of these synthetic drugs were developed by pharmaceutical companies, but discarded because their psychoactive effects were too powerful or other side-effects were considered too severe. In other cases, new synthetic psychoactive drugs are manufactured by modifying the chemical structure of existing drugs, in an attempt to make new and more powerful versions. For example, amphetamine, a stimulant drug, has been chemically modified to produce hundreds of similar drugs.

New synthetic drugs have been developed to mimic all the psychoactive drug effects a user could wish for, including synthetic stimulants, synthetic sedatives, synthetic hallucinogens and synthetic cannabis. There has never been a wider choice of drugs available to users. Many of these new variations fall outside existing drug control legislation and because of this are technically legal.

The rise of the synthetics

The past decade in particular has seen an extraordinary rise in the production and distribution of synthetic psychoactive drugs. Globally, 95 countries or territories have detected 541 new psychoactive substances since 2008 (United Nations Office on Drugs and Crime, 2013). There has been a huge increase in the number of new substances available for sale on European drug markets. Since 2008, that number has increased every year, with 101 new substances detected in 2014 alone (European Monitoring Centre for Drugs and Drug Addiction, 2015; Fig. 6.1).

One of the problems with the new synthetic drugs is that their effects can be much more powerful and unpredictable than the drugs they are trying to mimic. For example, some synthetic cannabinoids produce much stronger effects than natural cannabis. As the strength increases, so does the potential for harm, leading to problems such as rapid intoxication, abnormal heartbeat, psychosis and dependence syndrome.

So why do these drugs appeal to users? Surely they would prefer the more predicable, traditional drugs? Well, many

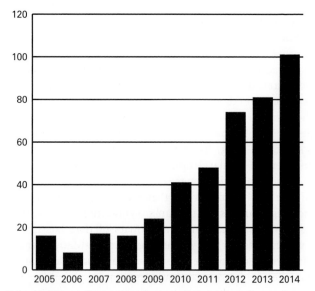

Fig. 6.1 Number of new synthetic psychoactive drugs detected in Europe each year.

do, but for certain groups of users, the newer drugs do hold some appeal. They are often more powerful, cheaper and easier to buy, so they attract people with not much money to spend. Many of the new drugs are still legal, an important consideration for people who don't want to risk a criminal record. Most of the drugs are so new that they are undetectable by standard drug testing. This may appeal to people who undergo regular drug testing in the workplace. As we can see, the new synthetic drugs have advantages over more traditional drugs for some groups of users. It is too early to say how these patterns of drug use will develop.

The world's biggest drug experiment

Perhaps the greatest risk of the new synthetic drugs is what we don't know about them. They are entirely untested. To understand this risk, let's look at the process of developing a new medication. All new medicines have to complete rigorous safety testing before they can be licensed for human use. Tests are conducted to look for immediate side-effects (e.g. rashes, bleeding) as well as harm caused by prolonged use (e.g. cancer, dementia). This extensive testing aims to spot drugs with unwanted or unpredictable effects and stop development before they are used by humans.

Safety testing has steadily improved over the decades, prompted by repeated medical disasters caused by medications reaching commercial markets only to later prove harmful. Thalidomide is a tragic example of the sort of harm that rigorous modern testing aims to prevent. Developed in the 1950s, thalidomide was thought to be so safe that it was prescribed to relieve anxiety and morning sickness in pregnancy. It was only later that the catastrophic harm it caused to unborn babies was detected.

The newly synthesised drugs have not been through any such rigorous testing. The short- and long-term health risks remain completely unknown. Users of these new synthetic drugs are essentially entering themselves into a huge, unregulated global drug trial, in which they are the guinea pigs. Unfortunately, in this unregulated, global 'trial', users will only know about a drug's problems when they experience the harm themselves.

The manufacturers and distributors of these new synthetic drugs are only too happy for users to act as their laboratory rats. Driven by profit, manufacturers have such a wide range of new synthetic drugs to choose from that they can afford to market and distribute large numbers and see which ones become popular. If users experience harm or even death, that drug is simply discarded as not profitable.

Legal but not safe

The term 'legal high' has been widely used to describe this group of synthetic drugs. Many of the new chemical structures are not directly mentioned in existing drug legislation and are therefore technically legal, despite being powerful drugs. Sellers often label these products 'not for human consumption', while at the same time making it clear how they can be used for exactly that purpose. In fact, the term legal high is misleading, as many of these products are actually blends of legal and illegal drugs and can be not only stimulating but also sedative, hallucinogenic and dissociative. In other words, legal highs are not always legal and don't always get you high.

Examples of legal high packaging are shown in the colour section. Many new synthetic drugs are available in head shops, which sell drug paraphernalia such as cigarette papers, bongs and herbal products. In some countries, the trade has spread to petrol stations and newsagents! As the number of new synthetic drugs has rapidly increased, the legal high traders needed a distribution network that was more accessible to users, was sheltered from potential prosecution, and where the products, if banned or found to be unsafe, could be rapidly replaced with new ones.

The role of the internet

As the trade in new synthetic drugs develops, the internet has become a key tool for promotion, sale and distribution. The number of online head shops selling cheap, potent drugs in the EU increased almost fourfold over only 4 years (European Monitoring Centre for Drugs and Drug Addiction, 2014). Delivery by post presents a huge challenge to law enforcement agencies and, in any case, selling psychoactive drugs that are not regulated by the 1971 United Nations Convention on Psychotropic Substances or subsequent legislation is not against the law.

For users, the internet is an attractive way to buy drugs. Rather than finding a dealer, with all the potential risk that can bring, users can now go online and with a few clicks of the mouse and a valid bank card, have a package of legal drugs delivered the very next day. The accessibility and legality of these new drugs has reportedly attracted new users, such as young professionals, who might previously not have considered using drugs for fear of getting caught, mixing with drug dealers or taking something they know can cause harm. However, many seem happy to try something that, without information to suggest otherwise, they believe is safe. As one of my patients said to me, 'It would be banned if it was dangerous, wouldn't it?'

From surface to dark web

Illegal drug dealers have also caught on to the internet as a way to cheaply distribute drugs. As well as online legal high sites, there are other ways to buy both legal and illegal drugs.

The internet can be considered as having three parts. The first is the surface web. This is the part that can be reached using popular search engines such as Google or Yahoo. These search engines work by identifying links, which are essentially anything you can click on.

The second part of the internet is known as the deep web. The content in this part cannot be reached by simply clicking on a link. Instead, tools such as search boxes are needed to access particular pages. Much of the internet's content is in the deep web and the content of these pages is usually legal, helpful and legitimate.

The final part of the internet is the dark web. This is a part of the deep web that has been intentionally hidden and can only be accessed with a certain amount of technical knowledge. A good way to visualise the web is to picture an iceberg: the surface web is what you can see above the water, the deep web is the larger part under the surface, and the dark web, at the very bottom, is almost invisible and difficult to get to (Fig. 6.2).

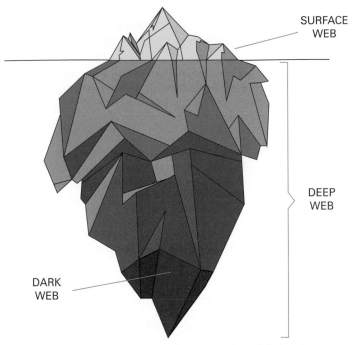

Fig. 6.2   The internet's surface web, deep web and dark web.

Online drug markets: the Silk Road

The dark web has recently become a serious concern for law enforcement agencies across the world. It has become the location for criminal activity, including the selling of illicit drugs. The most well known part of the dark web is TOR, previously known as The Onion Router. This describes the layers of encryption protecting a site that need to be peeled away before reaching the centre. This encryption allows users to be anonymous and untraceable. TOR can only be accessed using a specialist TOR web browser. The most well-known service on TOR was the Silk Road, an online marketplace through which users could anonymously buy almost anything using an online peer-to-peer currency known as bitcoins. In 2013, it was estimated that 70% of products sold on the Silk Road were psychoactive drugs (Ball, 2013). Drug dealers had discovered a new way to sell not only legal highs but also illegal drugs such as heroin and cocaine. In October 2013, the FBI closed down the Silk Road and arrested its founder (Taylor, 2015), but within a few months other TOR-supported sites sprang up in its place.

Online pharmacies

More recently, legal medicines with misuse potential, such as diazepam and codeine, have also been openly sold in 'online pharmacies'. These are often real medications sold through legitimate online pharmacies, but without the need for a prescription. In other cases they are counterfeit medications, chemical duds with no psychoactive effects, sold in a cynical attempt to make money.

New generation, new challenges

Synthetic psychoactive drugs, as with all psychoactive drugs, are most popular in younger age groups. This younger generation has grown up using the internet for almost every aspect of daily life, from buying a cinema ticket to running their social lives. What will be the effects of having powerful drugs easily available at the click of a mouse? Only by monitoring this emerging online drug distribution network will we find out.

It would be easy to see the internet as a threatening new tool for drug dealers, but it is also an important source of health information that is accessed and valued by young people (European Commission, 2014). There is a huge range of information on the internet about drugs, ranging from government-run information websites to user forums reviewing the latest novel psychoactive substances. Although the internet brings new challenges, it has huge potential to deliver accurate information about health risks. The Appendix lists useful resources.

Meeting the challenge: a game of cat and mouse

As the harm related to particular legal highs becomes evident, governments have moved to ban them. In many countries, there are rigorous processes to assess and consider banning new drugs. The first step in this process is to establish the level of harm a new drug is causing. A detailed, expert review of the evidence is conducted to work out how dangerous the new drug is likely to be to users. Based on this review, a decision is made whether to ban the substance. This process of careful scientific review can take several months.

Previously, new drugs only occasionally appeared on the drug market. Assessing harm and then deciding whether the harm is great enough to ban the drug worked well. But now the huge number of new psychoactive substances has overwhelmed the tried and tested process. There are two particular problems for regulators.

First, the sheer number of new substances is too much for the current system of careful review to cope with. Governments have previously assessed a handful of new substances a year. Now there might be a new substance every week. The system was simply not designed for this volume of work.

Second, a psychoactive substance is typically banned when there is clear evidence that it is likely to cause harm. This sensible and logical approach needs experts to carefully examine the research and gather expert opinion to build an accurate picture of the risks. There are many sources of information, ranging from academic literature to analysis of police seizures. However, there are now so many new psychoactive substances that for most of them, there is little or no evidence to examine. In many cases, the substances are simply too new for there to be helpful information to decide if they are safe or not.

To ban or not to ban

This is a real challenge for regulators. Do they wait for users to experience significant harm or even death, or do they ban a new drug without any evidence of problems? To further complicate matters, sometimes banning a drug actually increases its popularity, as some users seek it out for its notoriety.

As the problem of new psychoactive substances escalates, different countries are trying different approaches. Some have imposed blanket bans on vendors, while others have considered establishing a regulated market in which manufacturers of synthetic drugs need to prove the safety of their product before being given a licence to manufacture and sell it. The rise of synthetic drugs is too recent to be able to predict what will happen next, either in terms of their popularity or the effects of different methods of regulation. It is, however, likely that new, potent psychoactive drugs, with unknown risks, will continue to be easily accessible for the foreseeable future.

Key messages

- A huge number of new psychoactive substances have been marketed in the past decade, with more than 500 new drugs detected worldwide since 2008.

- These drugs are designed and marketed to mimic the effects of traditional drugs such as cocaine, heroin and cannabis.

- The new drugs are typically cheap and powerful and cause harm similar to (and sometimes more severe than) that of the drugs they mimic.

- Online sites are used to promote and sell newer drugs to younger audiences accustomed to the internet.

- Novel psychoactive substances challenge law enforcement and health systems in a manner not previously seen. The sheer number of new chemicals makes it difficult for existing systems of regulation and health professionals to keep up.

Detecting drug use and what to do about it

Chapter 3 looked at how you might talk to your child about drugs before they come into contact with them. But what if you think your child is actually using drugs?

How parents react to finding out their child is using drugs depends on the situation. There is a big difference between a child who experiments once or twice with cannabis before deciding it is not for them and a child who uses cocaine heavily, leading to major health problems. What is the best approach to take? Should you gently engage or directly confront them?

There is very little research in this area to draw on. Situations and families are so different that there is no guaranteed 'best' approach. The following suggestions are based on what has worked for the families I've encountered over my years in clinical practice.

What is normal adolescent behaviour?

Adolescence is a time of huge physical and psychological change. Many of these changes can confuse and worry parents. In most cases, the things parents see are completely normal parts of the process of growing up. However, a complication is that many of the normal signs of adolescence can mimic the signs of harmful drug use. Telling the difference can be virtually impossible without further information. Table 7.1 shows some of the overlap between the changes typical for puberty and the signs of drug use.

Given this overlap, how can you tell what's normal and what isn't? If your previously delightful and obedient child turns into a moody, irritable and withdrawn adolescent, should you assume it's because of hormones, or should you wonder whether they are using drugs?

Table 7.1 Comparing signs of puberty with signs of harmful drug use

Signs of puberty	Signs of possible drug use
Physical	
Acne or poor skin	Acne or poor skin
Reduced self-care and hygiene	Reduced self-care and hygiene
Excessive or poor sleep	Excessive or poor sleep
Change in energy levels	Change in energy levels
Rapid growth	Looks unwell
Change in appearance	Unexpected weight change
Body odour	Drug-specific signs: sores around mouth or nose (inhaling or snorting), conjunctivitis ('red eyes' with cannabis), injection marks (injecting)
Psychological	
Irritability and anger	Irritability and anger
Emotional withdrawal	Emotional withdrawal
Moodiness	Moodiness
Distractibility	Distractibility Unpredictable behaviour Self-harm (e.g. burning, cutting)[a]
Social	
Change in peer group	Change in peer group, particularly associating with people who use drugs
Experimentation with new fashions	Experimentation with new fashions, particularly with drug-related culture
Social withdrawal	Social withdrawal Too much or too little money (compared with what they should have) Significant, unexplained deterioration in academic performance Talking about drugs on social media Not being where they say they will be Paraphernalia of drug use (e.g. cigarette paper, bongs, straws for snorting)

a. This is also a feature of other emotional problems.

How to tell whether your child is using drugs

Most parents assume their children don't use drugs, and most children don't. However, UK statistics from 2013–2014 suggest that about a third of people between 16 and 24 years of age have taken an illicit drug at some point, equivalent to around 2.2 million young adults (Home Office, 2014).

If your child uses a drug once or twice at a party and then stops, you will probably never know, unless they decide to tell you or experience a bad reaction. If, on the other hand, your child starts to use regularly, you will probably start to notice changes in the way they look and behave.

How easy is it to detect drug use? It depends very much on the pattern of use. Let's use the examples of Andy and Alex.

Andy's story

Andy is a 16-year-old boy who has just finished his exams. He thinks he has done well and plans to return to school after the summer to study sciences at a senior level. With his exams over, Andy went camping with his school friends for a week. One of his friends brought some cannabis and over the week, Andy smoked six joints and drank a large amount of alcohol around a bonfire they made each night. Andy quite enjoyed the experience of smoking cannabis, particularly its relaxing effect. He did not experience any problems. On returning from his holiday, Andy made no attempt to buy cannabis and told his friends that he could 'take it or leave it'. Secretly, Andy is a bit worried about using something illegal and prefers getting drunk on alcohol in any case. Since then, he has not used any drugs.

Alex's story

Alex is also 16 years old and is in Andy's class, although not a close friend. He also intends to study science and, to celebrate the end of his exams, went away with a different group of friends to a large music festival near London. Before leaving for the festival, Alex, who had never used drugs before, decided that he was going to try ecstasy as a 'rite of passage'. He and his friends easily found a dealer at the festival. Alex had researched ecstasy on the internet. He was expecting a powder that he had planned to dab on his gum in small amount to see if he liked it. Instead, because he and his friends were sold tablets, they took one each and headed for the dance tent.

Alex had a 'brilliant night' and really enjoyed the effects of the tablet. He was still dancing at 6 am the next morning, and then became overwhelmed by tiredness and headed back to his tent to sleep.

The next evening, Alex was keen to try more ecstasy and asked his friends to come with him to find the dealer. His friends were not so keen. They felt exhausted, washed out and refused to go. Undeterred, Alex found the dealer again and this time bought two pills, which he took that evening. Alex had another 'great night' but the effects of the drugs were not quite as good as the night before. By the morning he was feeling ill with exhaustion and left the festival early to go home and rest. His friends stayed on for the last day.

Arriving home, Alex went to bed and slept for 16 hours. The next day his parents were troubled by his lack of energy, irritability and moodiness. Alex said that he was just tired from the festival. Later that week, Alex was still acting out of character, so his parents asked his friends if there had been any problems during the weekend. They said it had been the best weekend of their lives and that Alex had been on top form.

It took Alex nearly a week to feel back to normal after using ecstasy and he was surprised by how unwell he felt. Although pleased that he had tried the drug, he decided to avoid it for a while. But later that month, recalling the 'amazing' night he had at the festival, he began using ecstasy again.

It is unlikely that Andy's parents will ever know about his cannabis use unless he chooses to tell them. He seems to have experienced no lasting harm. Alex's parents, on the other hand, noticed that he was not himself and are likely to notice a similar change in behaviour if Alex continues to use ecstasy. The pattern of drug use will determine the probable harm, and it is the harm you are most likely to notice.

There are many ways you might find out that your child is using drugs. Here are some of the more common ones.

They tell you

Your child might try a drug and feel unwell. Worried, they might need advice and reassurance and turn to you for help. They are more likely to approach you if you have already talked about drugs with them (see Chapter 3).

Occasionally, children tell their parents about drug use as an aggressive and provocative act. If you think this is the case, consult a professional as, in my experience, there will usually be a number of complex issues to deal with.

Someone else tells you

Parents sometimes learn from others about their child's drug use: a concerned friend, another parent, a teacher at school or, more alarmingly, the police when they arrive on your doorstep having arrested or cautioned your child. Worse still, you might receive a call from a hospital department, saying that your child has collapsed and needed treatment.

Your child's friends, particularly those who don't use drugs, will often worry if they see a friend suffering as a result of their drug use. Without experience in managing these situations and anxious about getting their friend in trouble, they often don't know what to do. They may speak to their own parents, who in turn may speak to you or to a teacher at school. I have met many parents who are aware of another child's drug use but are not sure whether to speak to the child's parents or not. There is no right or wrong answer to this dilemma, but most parents would prefer to know if their child were using drugs, however upsetting finding out might be.

You see them intoxicated, or see the after-effects of drug use

If your child has taken a drug, they may return home from a night out clearly intoxicated. As described in Chapter 5, psychoactive drugs can be broadly categorised as stimulant, sedative, hallucinogen or dissociative agents and the effects of intoxication usually correspond to these descriptions (Table 7.2).

Some effects are common to all four groups. Mood can change rapidly, for example from happy and giggly to irritable and angry. Alcohol intoxication can also mimic many of the signs of drug use. People often use more than one drug at the same time, including alcohol, leading to a mixture of symptoms.

You find drugs or drug paraphernalia in their room

Parents sometimes find drugs or the paraphernalia of drug use (the equipment used to consume drugs) hidden in their child's bedroom or clothing. You might be unsure of exactly what you have found. Drugs are distributed and sold in a wide

Table 7.2 Common features of intoxication for different drug groups

Drug group	Common drugs	Features of intoxication
Stimulants	Cocaine, mephedrone, amphetamines, ecstasy	Alert, restless, agitated, euphoric, giggly, irritable, talking too quickly, distractible, aggressive
Sedatives	Alcohol, cannabis, heroin, benzodiazepines, GHB/GBL	Slurred speech, unsteady when walking, tired or sleepy, giggly, disinhibited, alcohol can be smelt on the breath
Hallucinogens	LSD, new synthetic hallucinogens, magic mushrooms	Distractible, responding to things that are not there, confused, frightened without apparent reason, paranoid
Dissociatives	Ketamine, nitrous oxide	Disorientated, uncoordinated, trance-like state

variety of forms and packaging. Some drugs are packaged in small, clear, resealable plastic bags, while others will be sold in brightly coloured foil, often with logos or branding. See the colour section for examples of common packaging.

Drugs can come in powder form: sometimes fine, sometimes crystalline and usually white. A white powder could be any of a wide range of drugs, including mephedrone, cocaine, ketamine, heroin, crushed-up medication or one of the many novel psychoactive substances now easily available.

Other drugs look like plant material, resin, tablets, capsules or blotting paper. Cannabis is usually easily identified as greenish-brown plant material. If you do find a drug in your child's room and don't know what it is, consider having it tested. Identifying the drug is very helpful in understanding the potential harm and what the next step might be.

Drug paraphernalia might give a clue about what drug is being used. Cigarette papers (a common brand is Rizla), pipes or bongs are commonly used to smoke cannabis, and powders are usually snorted using a mirror, straw and something to separate (chop) powder into a line. Small, silver, metal canisters, known as whippets, contain nitrous oxide. Syringes, needles or vials labelled 'water for injection' suggest that a drug is being injected and are clearly a very worrying sign.

Sometimes suspicion is raised by finding not drug paraphernalia but other, associated items. Clothing, bracelets and necklaces with a cannabis leaf symbol are common, but adolescence is a period of pushing boundaries and provocative clothing is often part of this. A Bob Marley poster appearing on a bedroom wall should not immediately lead to accusations of drug use! It might, however, be a useful way to open a conversation about drugs, if you have not yet done this.

Key messages

- Detecting drug use in adolescents can be difficult, as puberty can mimic many of the physical and emotional warning signs of drug use.
- It is important to be vigilant, but don't suggest your child is using drugs unless you have good reason to think so.

What to do if you know or suspect your child is using drugs

As we've seen, drug use is common, and it's more common in adolescents and young adults than in any other age group. Most people who use drugs do so for a short period and then stop, and most people do not experience significant harm unless their use increases.

In this context, let's think about your child. You suspect they're using drugs but are not sure. This suspicion may be based on indirect evidence, such as significant changes in behaviour or academic performance, or you may have seen them intoxicated or found drug paraphernalia in their room.

Believing your child is using drugs is usually very worrying. Not knowing for sure can raise all sorts of fears and as long as the situation is unclear it can be hard to know what to do. The steps listed next will help you understand the situation and decide what to do next.

Why are you suspicious?

It is important to understand the reasons for your concern and to think whether there are other explanations. If an adolescent is irritable, moody, withdrawn, and wearing a T-shirt with a cannabis leaf on it, it does not necessarily mean they are using drugs. There are other possibilities. Could it be the emotional rollercoaster of puberty, have they just argued with their best friend, are they struggling academically at school, or could they be depressed?

Act as a team

Share your concerns with people you trust. This could be your child's other parent or, depending on your circumstances, your current partner or a close friend. It is generally helpful to agree a way forward and act as a team. Sometimes the problem is only just beginning, and being a united team, supporting each other, will be important for both you and your child.

Being a parent is mostly a wonderful experience, but there are points when it can be very challenging. If you have just discovered that your child is using drugs, then you may be at one of those particularly challenging periods. It will be easier if you are not dealing with it on your own.

Talk to your child

If you suspect your child is using drugs, even if you think it's harmless experimentation, talk to them. If you don't ask, you miss giving them an opportunity to tell you. Explain that you are concerned about them and that you think they might be using drugs. It is sometimes helpful to say that, in your experience, drugs are sometimes used to cope with difficult feelings but that it is better to deal with those feelings rather than try to blot them out with drugs.

Accusing your child and putting them on the spot with a direct 'Are you using drugs?' question is too confrontational for the first conversation, unless you have clear evidence of drug use, such as finding drugs in their room. Explain that this is not a one-off conversation and that you want to help them if they will let you. Give them a chance to speak. They might respond with a wave of denials, or they might be relieved that they can finally tell you about it. Either way, your child now knows that you are aware of possible drug use and this might influence their future choices.

Talk to others

It is often helpful to talk to others. Discreetly asking the school if they have academic or pastoral concerns may give other clues as to what is going on. It might be helpful to talk to family members, friends your child spends time with, or staff at after-school activities your child attends.

Consider drug testing

This will be covered in detail later in the next section of this chapter.

Seek professional help if needed

When a child experiments with drugs, it can cause great distress and anguish for parents. Fortunately, most drug use and related behaviour turn out to be a brief episode in the child's journey to adulthood. Although this can be traumatic for parents, solutions are often reached without the need for outside help.

In other cases, however, professional help is needed. This could be your local family doctor, drug service or adolescent service. Sometimes the family is not in a position to successfully communicate with each other or agree a way forward. Parents sometimes need an independent opinion to reassure them that they are doing the right thing. In other cases, the child asks to talk to someone outside the family. Occasionally, things get so bad that the child's behaviour puts them or others in danger.

I suggest you seek professional help in any of the following circumstances:

- Your child is injecting or you suspect they're injecting any drugs.
- Suspected or confirmed use of a Class A drug.
- Your child asks to speak to a professional.
- Suicidal thinking or repeated self-harm (e.g. cutting, burning).
- Symptoms suggesting psychosis (e.g. intense paranoia, hearing voices, odd beliefs, bizarre behaviour).

- Your child places themselves at risk (e.g. sexual promiscuity, driving when intoxicated).
- Physical violence (actual or reported).
- Existing mental health problems (e.g. depression, anxiety).
- Previous drug or alcohol problems suggesting a repeating pattern of harmful use.
- Strong family history of addiction (e.g. close relative with a history of alcohol or drug problem).
- Parents are unable to successfully communicate with their child about what is going on.
- Rapid deterioration in academic, social or emotional functioning (e.g. deteriorating self-care, isolating themselves, refusing to attend school).

If any of the above describes your current situation, I strongly suggest you seek professional help. Many of these situations are associated with significant risk and need urgent assessment and management. There are many types of professional help available. Chapter 8 will look at different types of treatment and recovery services and what you can expect if you ask for professional help.

Key messages

If your child is using psychoactive drugs

- Talk to your partner, close friends or family
- Act as a team
- Talk to others – the school, people who know your child well
- Consider drug testing
- Seek professional help if the situation is deteriorating

Drug testing

To many parents, drug testing is seen as an independent, objective way of finding out if their child is using drugs. The reality of drug testing is a little more complicated. At best, drug testing is a tool to help understand what is going on and support treatment planning. It is not a treatment itself or a substitute for talking with your child, however difficult that conversation might be.

There are now many relatively cheap and accurate commercial tests available. Commercial drug tests usually use urine, saliva or hair samples, although blood-based testing is also possible. Each approach involves a different way of collecting the sample and a different level of accuracy.

Measuring recent or long-term use

Measuring recent use: urine, saliva and blood tests

Urine, saliva and blood samples can be tested for recent drug use, which usually means the past few days. The body excretes drugs at different speeds depending on the properties of the drug. Cannabis can stay in the body for several weeks, whereas stimulants such as cocaine are excreted much faster and may be undetectable after a few days. Once the sample is collected, some drug-testing kits need to be sent back to the manufacturer for analysis. Others provide on-the-spot results, similar to a pregnancy test.

Measuring long-term use: hair tests

It is sometimes important to know the longer-term pattern of use, rather than what has been used in the past few days. To examine drug use over longer periods, strands of hair can be tested. Some drugs and their metabolites can be detected in strands of hair for up to 90 days after use, using laboratory analysis. (When a drug is processed by the body, it is broken down to its chemical building blocks, called metabolites.) The sample is usually a strand of head hair of about 4 cm in length (1.5 inches), which is sent to the manufacturer for analysis. Results are usually available within a week and provide a summary of drug use over a month or more. Hair analysis is not very useful for detecting very recent drug use, as it takes a few days for a drug or its by-products to become embedded in the hair.

Accuracy

All commercial drug-testing methods have high accuracy for the drugs they test for, but are not 100% accurate. In other words, although very accurate they can occasionally show drug use when no drugs have been taken, or no evidence of drug use when a drug has been consumed. Repeating the testing is the best way to allow for this. Individual manufacturers will always provide information on the test's accuracy.

What drugs can be tested for?

Most of the kits currently available test for a range of common drugs. A typical drug screen would include cannabis, heroin, amphetamines, cocaine, methadone and benzodiazepines. Single-drug tests, for example just for cocaine, can also be purchased. Tests for less common drugs such as novel psychoactive substances (the so-called legal highs) are not generally available, but many manufacturers are willing to test for them if contacted.

Practicalities and pitfalls of drug testing

If you want to drug test your child, you will need their agreement. It is important to be very clear with them what you intend to do. Are you going to collect saliva, urine or hair as the sample? Will it be a one-off test, or something that is repeated? If it is to be repeated, how often? Will the tests be taken regularly, for example every Monday morning, or instead be randomly administered? What are you going to test for? With all these options, it is sometimes helpful to seek the support of a professional who can act as an independent negotiator (see below).

There are several factors to consider when deciding to test your child for drugs.

What if your child refuses to take a drug test?

If your child refuses to take a drug test, there is little you can do other than assume they are using drugs. Trying to secretly take a sample from your child, however ingenious your plan, is not a good approach. To be useful, drug testing needs to be agreed by all sides.

Is it possible to cheat a drug test?

There are many ways to cheat a drug test. The simplest way is to avoid producing a genuine sample. Let's consider urine testing. Parents may be reluctant to intrude on their children's bathroom privacy. However, unless you know the urine has come directly from your child into the test container, you don't know if it has been substituted with something else – water from the tap, perhaps, or another person's urine. The only way to confirm that the sample is valid is by direct observation.

The easiest way to avoid giving a genuine sample is to use a sample from someone who has not consumed any drugs. For urine testing, this might involve using someone else's urine or buying synthetic urine on the internet. Most urine drug-testing kits have a temperature strip to check the sample is at body temperature. Substituted or synthetic urine, even if held close to the body, rarely reaches body temperature.

Another common technique is to dilute the urine, either by adding water to the sample or by drinking large quantities of water prior to the test. Most testing kits are able to detect drugs in very small qualities and dilution in this way usually does not work. It is important to examine the urine sample, however, to make sure it is not just water straight from the bathroom tap.

It is generally more straightforward to supervise the collection of the sample in saliva testing, although the technology is newer and less widely used.

An alternative to home testing is to have a specialist drug service or even your family doctor supervise the drug testing for you. This takes the pressure off parents to collect the sample and ensure it has been taken correctly.

When and how often will you administer a drug test?

Both parent and child must have a clear understanding of how often the drug testing will take place and whether it will be regular or random. Agreeing this with your child in advance reduces the chance of disagreement later on.

Which drugs to test for?

You may have a suspicion that your child is using a particular drug, for example cannabis, and feel that testing for cannabis alone will be sufficient. It is true that some people use just one drug. However, most people who use one drug experiment with several, often using more than one drug at a time and often combining them for particular effects. For example, a stimulant user may use a sedative at the end of the night to reduce the unwanted alertness and insomnia of the stimulant drug.

So, if you are going to test your child for drugs, it makes sense, at least initially, to test for a range of common drugs. Be aware that there are no commercially available home-based drug tests that will detect all drugs. The only way to test for all known drugs would be to send the sample to a specialist laboratory that would test the sample using an advanced analytical technique.

What will you do with the results?

It will be a huge relief for you if the result of a drug test is negative. There are, however, a few things to bear in mind. Drugs are detectable for only a short time in the blood, urine and saliva, and different drugs last for different lengths of time depending on the properties of the individual drug and the amount taken. Table 7.3 shows the typical length of time you would expect a urine or saliva test to be able to detect different drugs for after use (Department of Health, 2007; Australian National Council on Drugs, 2013). Hair testing can detect most drugs for up to a month after use.

However, if the drug test detects one or more drugs, then what? In this situation, you need to sit down with your child and see if you can agree a plan. They may admit that they have been using drugs, but sometimes they will be adamant that they have taken nothing. Remember, drug tests can return false

Table 7.3 How long after use various drugs can be detected by testing urine or saliva

Drug	Saliva test (at home)	Saliva test (sent to lab)	Urine test (at home)	Urine test (sent to lab)
Cannabis (occasional use)	<24h	<24h	<10 days	<10 days
Cannabis (chronic use)	<24h	<24h	≥30 days	≥30 days
Cocaine	<24h	<3 days	2–3 days	2–3 days
Opioids	<24h	<3 days	2–4 days	2–4 days
Amphetamines	<24h	<3 days	2–5 days	<14 days
Methamphetamines	<24h	<3 days	2–5 days	2–5 days
Benzodiazepines	<24h	<3 days	<14 days	<14 days

Sources: Department of Health (2007), Australian National Council on Drugs (2013).

positive results, which means they might be telling the truth. The best thing to do in this case is to repeat the test as soon as possible. If the second test also detects drugs, then it is highly likely that there are drugs in their body.

You may ask them to stop using drugs and, if they agree, suggest repeating the drug test in a week or so. If they continue to say they haven't used drugs or refuse to stop using, then it is probably time to seek professional help.

Drug testing is not a foolproof way to find out if your child has taken drugs. It might be a useful tool in helping you understand whether your child is experiencing drug-related problems and may also be a useful part of a treatment plan, but it is no substitute for an open dialogue with your child.

Key messages

- Drug testing can be helpful, but it is not a treatment or a substitute for talking with your child.

- If you decide to test your child for drugs, it is crucial that you agree with them what is going to happen.

- Recent drug use (over the last few days) can be tested using urine, saliva or blood. Longer term drug use (over the last month) can be tested using strands of hair.

- Most drug tests will only detect commonly used drugs such as cocaine and cannabis. Tests for novel psychoactive substances (so-called legal highs) are not routinely available. Talk to the manufacturer if you want to test for newer drugs.

- No drug test is 100% accurate. Repeating drug testing reduces the risk of false results.

- There are many ways to cheat a drug test. The only way to be sure of the source of a sample is to be present while it's taken.

Treatment and recovery

So far, this book has focused on the problems different drugs cause. It is now time to look at how to tackle these problems. This chapter will look at what treatments are available, how well they work and what you and your child can expect from your treating team.

A challenging fact about drug problems is that, unlike most other health problems, not everyone who needs help, wants it. Knowing that you have a problem and wanting to recover is sometimes called having insight into the condition. People with drug problems sometimes have poor insight into their problems and need for help. This can make things very difficult for worried relatives and concerned clinicians.

Some people want treatment, others don't

Many people who come to my clinic are suffering terribly from the effects of using drugs and are desperate to stop, but struggling to do this. They ask for my help to stop the drug use and get their lives back on track. Motivated to change, they work hard to get better and tend to do well in treatment.

But not everyone wants treatment, or even accepts there is anything wrong. Young people are sometimes dragged to see me by their worried parents. They don't think they have a problem, don't want to make any changes to their drug use and are usually very clear that I'm wasting my time.

In my experience, it is very difficult to help someone who does not wish to change. The treatment of drug problems is very much a collaborative effort between the patient and their treating team, with relatives often very involved. If there is no cooperation, helping someone can be tough, and I find it particularly upsetting to see people deteriorate when treatment could help. However, there is usually little point in trying to strong-arm into treatment someone who doesn't want help at that moment. A better approach is often to help them reduce their current risks as much as possible and keep gently explaining that treatment might help – if only they would agree to try it. Circumstances can change rapidly and as harms develop, so can the realisation that things can't go on as they are. Sometimes, keeping the door open and waiting is a better option than trying to push someone through it when they have dug in their heels.

Another common challenge is when a drug user minimises their problems. Despite clear evidence that their drug use has spiralled out of control, the patient will say they want to 'cut down a bit'. Even if this seems unrealistic, it is better to begin by working towards that goal and agreeing to try something else if this approach doesn't work.

All treatment starts with a detailed assessment of the problem. The better the problem is understood, the more likely the best treatment will be found. No two patients are alike and every treatment plan should be individually tailored.

Defining the problem

Many people approaching treatment ask for help to stop using drugs, but some are less clear about what they want. Chapter 4 explained how the harm caused by drugs generally depends on the pattern of use: recreational, harmful or dependence. Drug treatment services usually begin by trying to understand which of these three categories best describes the patient's drug use. This requires an assessment of the patient's level of control over the problem substance. Can the person control when they start using a drug, when they stop and how much they use? Understanding the level of control is important because it helps define the problem and choose the best treatment.

Testing the level of control

To understand a person's level of control, the patient and clinician need to work together. The best approach is to jointly agree a test of control. Usually this is a reduction in drug use or a period of abstinence combined with careful monitoring. For example, a patient might agree a goal of stopping all drugs for 2 weeks. Another might agree to try using only at weekends or no more than a certain amount each day. The patient keeps a detailed 'consumption diary' – a record of any drug use along with a description of what happened if things did not go to plan. Were they able to keep to the target or was it too difficult?

This approach requires honest recording of drug use, and comes back to the collaborative nature of treatment. If a goal has been agreed beforehand by the patient, it is their goal, not one imposed by the clinician. The case study below illustrates the process.

Eddie's story

Eddie is a 17-year-old mephedrone user. Mephedrone is a synthetic stimulant used in clubs that gives the user increased energy, alertness and often feelings of euphoria. Eddie started using drugs when he was 14 years old and 'went a bit mad'. He did poorly in his school exams and, at 16, left home to live with friends. Although things have 'calmed down' with respect to other drugs and alcohol, Eddie is concerned about his mephedrone use.

Over the past 6 months, his mephedrone use has gradually crept up and he is now using the drug with his friends at clubs or house parties most weekends. Although he still has a 'great time', he is beginning to experience problems. The worst of these is depression lasting 3–4 days after a drug binge. Eddie knows that mephedrone is the cause but can't seem to stop using it.

When he first came to see me, Eddie had 'one question' and wanted help with 'one goal'. He wanted to know whether he was addicted to mephedrone and asked for help to use less, but not to stop. In other words, he wanted to better control his mephedrone use. During our meeting, Eddie set himself the goal of using only twice a month for the next 3 months and not to take more than 1 g each time. He agreed to keep an honest diary of what actually happened and to record any important feelings, such as cravings.

He returned 3 weeks later, saying the plan had been 'a disaster'. Rather than reducing his use as he had hoped, he had actually taken more mephedrone than usual, even using one Tuesday evening while on his own, something he had never done before. Eddie admitted that at his first appointment he had lied about how much mephedrone he was using because he was worried it would 'look bad'. He now agreed that he didn't know how to control the mephedrone and wanted to stop entirely.

Eddie was disappointed that he couldn't control his mephedrone use. He really wanted to keep using with his friends but only now and again. It was not until he tested his control that he realised he couldn't do it. Admitting this was difficult for Eddie, but by setting his own goals and not reaching them, he found it easier to accept the reality.

Since then, Eddie has regularly attended the clinic. He is popular with staff because of his sharp sense of humour. Working hard in treatment, Eddie has achieved his new goal and has stopped using all drugs. In particular, he has worked with our psychologist to learn ways of avoiding temptation and has also used the sessions to improve his relationship with his family.

At the time of writing, Eddie has not used drugs or alcohol for over a year, is studying again and describes life as 'pretty wonderful'.

Where to get help

There exists a wide variety of drug treatment and recovery services. They are provided by the government, charities, private organisations and volunteers. Some services are available only to people living close by, and others will accept anyone. Services can be very different and it can be confusing for parents to understand what different organisations can offer and their level of expertise.

In general, age determines the service. For those under 16 years of age, treatment is usually provided by child and adolescent mental health services or specialist young people's drug services. The transition to adult health services occurs between 16 and 21 years of age, depending on the service.

Drug services for those over 16 years of age can be divided into two types. The first type manages immediate and short-term medical and psychological problems. The second type, sometimes called rehabilitation and recovery services, focuses on longer-term psychological treatments to help people who have stopped using drugs from returning to them.

If you think your child needs either type of help, call or visit the service. Ask them how they work and whether they think they can help. Services should be able to explain the type of approach they would use and why, helping you to decide whether it is right for your child.

Immediate and short-term treatment services

These specialist services will help anyone, even if they don't want to stop using drugs, but just want some advice or help to use less. Referral is usually made from a family doctor or other health professional, although many services offer drop-in clinics, where patients or their families can attend without needing an appointment.

Specialist drug services are provided by a team. The team usually includes doctors (including psychiatrists), nurses, psychologists, family therapists, social workers, drug workers and peer mentors (people who have been through treatment themselves and now work in the service to help others). This range of skills is important – every person asking for help is unique and a team of experts can help with problems in different ways.

Medical and psychological treatments such as medically assisted detoxification, sometimes called 'detox', are offered. An addiction psychiatrist, or sometimes a GP with specialist training, will usually take overall responsibility for treatment, particularly for physical and mental health problems or any medication prescribed.

Psychological therapy is the 'golden thread' that runs through all drug treatment and is usually provided by psychologists, specialist nurses or other specifically trained health professionals. Length of treatment can vary greatly. Some people will attend only once for advice, others will have treatment lasting months.

Depending on the problem and what changes the patient wants to make, treatment can help the person stop using altogether (abstinence) or cut down (controlled use). Drug use can cause many different problems, so treatment needs to cover the patient's physical, psychological and social needs. Most important of all is finding out how they developed a drug problem in the first place. The answer or answers might help prevent further drug use.

Once specialist treatment is completed, people are often referred to longer-term services for further support. Rehabilitation and recovery services help people build on the gains made so far.

Rehabilitation and recovery services

Rehabilitation and recovery services provide longer-term psychological and social support and are mostly for people who have been diagnosed with dependence syndrome. They are usually targeted at people who want to stop using psychoactive substances for good. Referral to rehabilitation is usually made by a health professional but can sometimes be made directly by a family member or the person with the problem. Many rehabilitation services offer residential programmes in which people live on site, often for several months, while they have further intensive psychological treatments.

Other recovery services are run by volunteers. Alcoholics Anonymous, Cocaine Anonymous and Narcotics Anonymous are organisations that offer free support meetings for people who want to live life without any psychoactive substances. Importantly, they are run by people already in recovery. These anonymous meetings run on a 12-step approach and offer mentoring (Alcoholics Anonymous, 2015). Each of the steps helps develop the understanding and skills to maintain abstinence. They can be an extremely valuable recovery support.

Confidentiality

Unless your child is very young, it is likely that they will be offered some time on their own with staff while you wait outside. This is not compulsory and many children ask for their parents to be present throughout the assessment. If they do want to talk without you, however, this part of the assessment is confidential and it will be explained to your child that anything they say will not be shared with you (unless they want it to be). The exception is if the professional feels that your child poses a danger to themselves or others, in which case confidentiality may be broken. The General Medical Council (2007) has clear instructions for doctors regarding confidentiality for those under 18 years old.

Parents can sometimes, quite understandably, feel frustrated by this principle of confidentiality, especially as it does not work the other way round. The health professional may insist that anything you say to them will be shared with your child. However, the advantage of time alone with the health professional and the assurance of confidentiality is that your child can tell their story in a setting where they feel they can be entirely honest without damaging relationships with their family.

What to expect when seeing a professional

The purpose of meeting with a professional is for an expert view on what might be going on with your child and what can be done to help. This starts with a thorough assessment to understand the current problems in the context of your family.

Assessment

The assessment may be carried out by different members of the team and can take several meetings to complete. Building trust with your child is the first task and this can take time. The assessment will cover your child's current and past drug use (including alcohol) and try to understand their motivations for using drugs. This will include questions about any previous treatment for drug use, what worked and what didn't work. The assessment will also include questions on family history and psychological, physical and social issues, a physical examination and urine, saliva or blood tests.

Following assessment, the assessor will meet with you and your child to talk about possible ways forward. This is sometimes written down in the form of a care plan (or treatment agreement) that includes a list of agreed aims, tasks and timescales. Examples include your child keeping an accurate diary of their drug use. Often these 'consumption diaries' will help identify places, people or activities that seem to trigger the drug use. The assessment is designed to gather as much information as possible, so the team can build a picture of the factors influencing drug use behaviour.

Goal-setting

One of the key parts of planning treatment is goal-setting. Your child will be asked to identify changes that they want to make and to plan how they might achieve those changes. Often the professional will suggest goals. They will depend on the severity of the drug use (recreational, harmful or dependent use) and factors such as how the drug is taken (orally, nasally, injected), the social context and genetic history. The treatment goals should be SMART: simple, measurable, attainable, realistic and timely.

As mentioned already, it is crucial that the goals are agreed by your child. If your child does not freely agree to them, however sensible those goals may be, they need to be re-thought. I often see children reluctantly agreeing to goals identified, often forcefully, by their parents. The child believes the goals are unrealistic and leaves the assessment with no intention of even attempting to achieve them. When the goals are inevitably not met, you and your child might feel a powerful sense of failure and lose confidence in the treatment process.

A better approach is to set smaller, more realistic goals, even if initially they seem very modest. Parents can feel frustrated by this approach, as they want to see problems dealt with as quickly as possible. Frustration can also result from children setting goals that their parents don't agree with. A good example is reducing rather than stopping drug use. Most of the time, parents want their children to stop using drugs entirely. This is a very sensible goal, but the child may find the idea of giving up drugs forever difficult to imagine. They might feel trapped by their drug use and by the people they use drugs with. Abstinence can feel impossible ('All my friends use drugs, there is no way I can be with them and never use again.'). Unless your child feels ownership of the treatment goals, treatment is likely to be a battle against your child, rather than with them, and it is less likely to succeed.

Why are they using drugs?

Chapter 1 described two broad motivations for drug use: to experience new feelings and to take away unwanted feelings. An important part of the assessment is exploring the reasons for drug use. It is usually very hard for a person to reduce or stop their drug use if the reason they are using drugs in the first place is not addressed.

It can take the clinical team many meetings to understand these motivations and, as parents, you are likely to have a very important part to play. You know your child better than anyone and might have a good idea what the underlying problems are.

If you think you know why your child is using drugs, then share this with the team. The more information they have, the better they are able to help.

Key treatments and recovery interventions

Understanding the different treatment and recovery options can be bewildering. Many services use technical language or unfamiliar words to describe treatments, so if you are not sure what something means, always ask. As parents, you will often play a crucial part in the treatment, so you need to know what is going on.

There are three main types of treatment:

- pharmacological treatment (prescribing medication)
- psychological treatment (talking therapies)
- social intervention (changing the environment).

Box 8.1 lists examples of the different treatment approaches. Several treatments might be combined, depending on the problems and the treatment goals.

Box 8.1   Examples of drug treatments

Pharmacological treatments

- Detoxification (depending on drug)
- Maintenance (methadone, buprenorphine)
- Blockade (naltrexone)

Psychological treatments

- Brief intervention
- Motivational interventions
- Contingency management
- Behavioural couples therapy
- Relapse prevention
- Cognitive–behavioural therapy (often abbreviated as CBT) and psychodynamic therapy for associated mental health problems

Social treatments

- Narcotics Anonymous
- Cocaine Anonymous
- Education and back-to-work programmes

Pharmacological treatment

Pharmacological treatment involves the prescription of medication, and the choice of medication will depend on the reason for prescribing it.

Detoxification

- Some psychoactive drugs cause dependence. Once dependent, patients can experience unpleasant or even life-threatening withdrawal symptoms if they go without the drug.
- Detoxification (detox), also called medically assisted withdrawal, involves prescribing medication to help treat these withdrawal symptoms. Medications are continued until the withdrawal symptoms have completely stopped, which can sometimes take a week or more.
- Different drugs cause different withdrawal symptoms for different lengths of time. Therefore, medications prescribed for heroin withdrawal are not the same as those prescribed for cocaine.

Maintenance

- Once someone has stopped using a drug, there are medications that can help them stay off it. Medications can reduce the desire or cravings to use drugs and are taken every day for several months.
- Other medications work as a substitute for the drug. They work on the same brain receptors as the drug the person has stopped using, but cause less harm. An example is methadone, prescribed for heroin dependence. Methadone, like heroin, works on the brain's opioid receptors. Unlike heroin, however, it is pharmacologically pure, without any of the contaminants found in heroin, making it safer. As methadone is prescribed by the clinic, the patient no longer needs to go to a dealer to buy heroin. This can help break the cycle of use for many patients.
- Maintenance medications are always prescribed alongside psychological and social treatments and are helpful for people who are struggling to stop using drugs. They can be a first step from illegal drugs to safer, prescribed drugs, before stopping drugs altogether. Maintenance medications are only available for some drugs.

Blockade

- Some medications work by blocking the brain receptors where drugs act. This means that when a person uses a drug, they won't experience any psychoactive effects. These blocking medications are only available for some drugs.
- Many of the more recent drugs, such as the novel psychoactive drugs or so-called legal highs, currently have no available pharmacological treatments.

Psychological treatment

Psychological treatment involves talking about problems and is sometimes called talking therapy. Psychological treatment is based on theories of how to change behaviour. Treatment can be in groups with other patients or one-to-one with a therapist, and usually happens weekly or fortnightly.

Therapists' training can vary considerably. Some of the most highly trained therapists are psychologists. I recommend that you check which organisation a therapist is accredited by and what treatments they have been trained to deliver.

In the UK, the National Institute for Health and Care Excellence (2007b) has reviewed the effectivenesss of psychological treatments for drug-related problems.

Social intervention

Just as important as how drugs interact with the brain is what happens outside of the brain. Family interactions, the influence of peers, environmental stress and occupational roles all influence the likelihood of harmful drug use. Social interventions tackle the situational factors contributing to harmful drug use and encourage an environment in which sustained recovery is nurtured.

When a person has recovered from a drug problem, the support of other people who have experienced similar problems can be very helpful. As already discussed, Narcotics Anonymous and similar organisations offer free support groups, which are run by people who have experienced drug problems and are in recovery. As well as offering support to people with drug problems, they also support relatives. Al-Anon is the most widely available (www.al-anonuk.org.uk). Another peer-support organisation is SMART recovery (www.smartrecovery.

org.uk), which uses evidence-based motivational, behavioural and cognitive strategies to help people recover from drug use.

Employment, training and study give young people's lives stability and purpose. Drug treatment services help people access further training and education and support them to prepare and apply for work. This can be crucial in helping someone stop using drugs.

What if drugs are only part of the problem?

Some patients have more than just drug problems. It's common to see drug use and mental or physical health problems (comorbid problems) in the same person at the same time. Mental health problems could include depression or anxiety, whereas physical problems could include chronic pain.

Drug use can be caused by underlying problems. If these problems are not addressed, even the best treatment programme is likely to fail. For example, some adolescents who use drugs also experience psychological problems such as depression. They might be using the drugs as a way of coping with the negative feelings. If the depression is not treated, drug use is likely to continue. Cognitive–behavioural therapy is usually the first choice for treating depression, but antidepressants may be needed, particularly if the symptoms are severe or there is suicidal thinking. Evidence-based treatments for comorbid problems have been reviewed by the National Insitute for Care and Excellence (2011) in the UK.

How good is treatment? Will it help my child?

Can treatment lead to sustained change or just temporary improvement? Will it work for everyone? That depends on many things, including a person's motivation to change, which drugs they are using and what level of support they have from family and friends.

Most drug users under 18 years of age recover. Of nearly 20 000 UK young people in drug treatment in 2013–2014, 80% successfully completed it (Public Health England, 2015). Most were using cannabis and very few were injecting drugs.

For those 16–59 years of age, however, only about a third of people who began treatment after 2005 completed it and did not return (Public Health England, 2014). Why do adults do worse in treatment than younger people? There are several contributing factors. Adults tend to use more harmful drugs, like heroin, and are more likely to inject them. They have been taking drugs for longer and are more likely to be dependent. This in turn leads to physical and mental health problems and broken relationships with friends and family, all of which lessens the chance of treatment succeeding.

Achieving treatment success

Some clear messages emerge from looking at treatment success. Those who don't inject, avoid heroin and crack, enter treatment early and have supportive families and friends do better. Drug treatment can work, particularly when it focuses not just on drugs but on the reasons for drug use.

What to do if treatment is not helping?

Even with professional help, problems don't always improve and sometimes even get worse. Treatment can uncover unacknowledged difficulties (e.g. underlying mental health problems) that complicate recovery. Barriers to recovery, until tackled, will keep your child returning to harmful behaviours.

If you think treatment is not helping, it is always best to talk to the professional in charge of your child's care. They need as much information as possible if they are to build an accurate picture of your child's problems and offer the best help. Don't keep quiet if you think things aren't going well. Medication or therapy might need to be changed or psychological approaches delivered by someone with more experience.

Sustained recovery

The concept of recovery is broadly defined as:

> 'A process of change through which individuals improve their health and wellness, live a self-directed life, and strive to reach their full potential.' (Public Health England, 2014)

The majority of young people with drug problems, once they tackle the issue, will stop using drugs and move on with their lives. Others, particularly those with drug dependence, find their drug problems keep coming back. For this group, recovery is not a point reached when they are 'cured'. Instead, it is a life-long process of managing their vulnerability to drugs. In this way, they're similar to people with other long-term illnesses such as asthma, diabetes or high blood pressure. The underlying problem does not go away and needs to be carefully controlled to avoid the symptoms returning.

Tessa's story

Tessa is 14 years old. Everything is going wrong. Despite having a caring family, no history of trauma and attending a well-regarded local school, Tessa feels angry, lonely and sad. Without any reason to explain her feelings, Tessa feels confused, overwhelmed and distressed by a feeling of being 'sucked underground', and had started using drugs as a way of coping.

To begin with she used cannabis, but soon started taking amphetamines and things really went downhill from there. She lost her remaining friends, was failing at school and her behaviour at home became increasingly unpredictable and aggressive. Tessa's parents are at a loss. They have an older daughter, Fiona, who is flourishing and they cannot understand how their two children can be so different.

Tessa agrees to start treatment and it is immediately clear that she is clever and thoughtful but troubled. She enjoys taking drugs, saying that they 'make all the feeling go away. I get a break from my head'.

Over the next few months, I learn more about Tessa. She has very low self-esteem and cannot think of a single thing she is good at. Intimidated by her older sister's achievements, Tessa describes herself as the 'black sheep of the family', saying that at least this gives her a role. She isn't clinically depressed but there is a strong family history of alcohol and drug use. Both grandfathers and two aunts had needed treatment for addictions.

Over 6 months in treatment, Tessa makes significant progress. She has stopped using all drugs and is working hard in psychological therapy. The rest of her family comes to some of the sessions to talk about how they speak to each other. Tessa celebrates her 15th birthday and is confident enough to invite some of her classmates. Everything seems to be going to plan.

A few weeks later, I receive an urgent phone call. It is Tessa's mother, who has found cannabis in Tessa's bedroom. Tessa initially denied the cannabis is anything to do with her, but her mother, using some of the skills developed in the family sessions, encouraged her to be honest. Tessa soon admitted to using cannabis and amphetamines again.

When Tessa next comes to see me, she is very despondent. She had worked so hard the first time around that she doesn't know what else she can do. It feels like one more failure. Her parents also feel terribly disappointed.

Over the next 18 months, this pattern of making progress then suddenly slipping back repeats two more times. Each time, Tessa does very well in treatment before returning to chaotic use of cannabis and amphetamines. The strong family history suggests that there might be a genetic element to Tessa's drug use and I begin to talk to her about how she can break the cycle of relapse.

We work more intensively on her self-esteem and help her spot the signs of relapse. Tessa also begins attending groups run by people in recovery, which she finds very supportive. She is now meeting people who have achieved what she is trying to do: find a way to live life without drugs.

A few years pass, Tessa is now 19 years old and works in marketing, something she loves. Compared with the sad, angry 14-year-old I first met, she is now a bright, confident young adult with a wonderful sense of humour. She hasn't used drugs for more than 2 years but describes herself as an addict. She thinks of her 'addiction' as a life-long problem that needs careful monitoring to keep it in check.

She says that her brain is 'wired' in a way that means she has no control over drugs. Over time, she has become very skilled at spotting the warning signs of relapse and has many psychological tools to manage high-risk situations and periods of stress. Tessa continues to regularly meet with other people in recovery and also drops by to see me a few times a year for a check-up.

When I meet with Tessa now, she no longer talks much about managing drug problems. Instead, she speaks about her career and hopes for the future. It has taken 5 years of ups and downs to get to this point, but all the hard work was worth it.

Key messages

- There are many different treatments and recovery services available. The best ones combine psychological treatment, social intervention and (where appropriate) medication.

- Ask services to explain the treatments they think will work for your child.

- The better the service understands your child, the better they will be able to help. Share all the information you have.

- It is important that your child can be open and honest with the professionals. This may mean that not everything is shared with you.

Final thoughts

This book is my way of sharing two decades of experience in helping people with drug problems. Using the latest science on how drugs work in the brain, I have tried to show their attraction as well as the problems they cause. Drug use peaks in adolescence, just at the time when the developing brain is uniquely vulnerable to their harmful effects.

For parents with children who are not using drugs, I hope the advice in this book will help stop problems developing. Having the drug conversation with your child before they are exposed to drugs will allow you to return to the topic if needed, without your child fearing that you are unable or unwilling to discuss it. They may then come to you earlier and be more honest about drugs, giving you a better chance of helping.

For parents with children who are experiencing drug problems, I hope this book has provided useful advice and either reassured you that you are doing the right things or helped you see a new path. There are no easy solutions and no simple right or wrong approaches. Much will depend on your relationship with your child and working as a team with family and friends.

I will finish with the key messages that, in my experience, parents have found helpful.

Preventing drug use

Start early

Try to have a knowledgeable, open conversation about drugs before your child is exposed to them or people using them.

Provide accurate information

Make sure your child knows where to get reliable information and is aware of any specific vulnerabilities they have to drugs, such as family history.

Remain vigilant

Your child will almost certainly be offered drugs at some point and may or may not try them. Adolescence is a difficult period, during which huge physical, psychological and social changes take place. Be vigilant for changes that might suggest that your child is coming into contact with drugs, for example changes in peer groups or academic performance.

Managing drug use

Is there a problem?

If you think your child is using drugs, try to establish what is really going on. This will almost certainly involve you speaking to them and perhaps others.

Stay calm

Most children who use drugs will moderate or stop their use of their own accord.

Find out what the underlying problem is

If your child is using drugs, why now? What is your child getting out of it? Does it give them exciting new feelings? Take away unwanted feelings? Are they trying to fit in with a particular social group? The better you understand their motivations for use, the better equipped you will be to help.

Get help

If behaviours are becoming too difficult to manage, it is time to seek professional help. Drug treatment works, and if your child needs help they should receive treatment, just as with any other health problem.

Look after yourself

There are few situations more stressful that seeing your child's physical, psychological and social health deteriorate as they use drugs. You might be tempted to downplay your own feelings, but it is important that you look after yourself. You will be better able to help your child if you have a clear plan and look after your own health. Use your social support, such as family or friends, and if this is not enough, seek professional help yourself.

Appendix

Drug information

National Institute for Health and Care Excellence
www.nice.org.uk
Offers a range of guidance for medical professionalson drug and alcohol problems

Talk to Frank
www.talktofrank.com
Government drug-information website for England and Wales

Know the Score
http://knowthescore.info
Government drug-information website for Scotland

National Institute on Drug Abuse
www.drugabuse.gov
Government drug-information website for the USA

DrugScience
www.drugscience.org.uk
Independent drug-information website

Crew 2000
www.crew2000.org.uk
Independent drug-information website for Scotland

Angelus Foundation
www.angelusfoundation.com
Independent website about 'legal highs' for adolescents

Alcohol Concern
www.alcoholconcern.org.uk
Independent alcohol-information website for the UK

NEPTUNE
www.neptune-clinical-guidance.co.uk
Independent website with guidance for clinicians on club drugs

Finding help

NHS Choices
www.nhs.uk/Livewell/drugs/Pages/Drugshome.aspx

Narcotics Anonymous
www.ukna.org

Cocaine Anonymous
www.cauk.org.uk

Alcoholics Anonymous
www.alcoholics-anonymous.org.uk

Marijuana Anonymous
www.marijuana-anonymous.co.uk

SMART Recovery
www.smartrecovery.org.uk

Support for families

Al-Anon
www.al-anonuk.org.uk

Adfam
www.adfam.org.uk

Professional bodies

Royal College of Psychiatrists, Faculty of Addictions Psychiatry
www.rcpsych.ac.uk/workinpsychiatry/faculties/addictions.
aspx

British Psychological Society, DCP Faculty of Addictions
www.bps.org.uk/networks-and-communities/member-microsite/dcp-faculty-addictions

British Association of Social Workers, Alcohol and Other Drugs Special Interest Group
www.basw.co.uk/group/?id=10

References

Action on Addiction (2013) *The Management of Pain in People with a Past or Current History of Addiction*. Action on Addiction.

Advisory Council on the Misuse of Drugs (2015) *Prevention of Drug and Alcohol Dependence – Summary*. ACMD.

Agrawal A, Lynskey MT (2006) The genetic epidemiology of cannabis use, abuse and dependence. *Addiction*, **101**, 801–12.

Agrawal PR, Scarabelli TM, Saravolatz L, *et al* (2015) *Current strategies in the evaluation and management of cocaine-induced chest pain*. Cardiology in Review, 23, 303–11.

Alcoholics Anonymous (2015) *The Twelve Steps of Alcoholics Anonymous*. AA (http://www.alcoholics-anonymous.org.uk/About-AA/The-12-Steps-of-AA).

Australian National Council on Drugs (2013) *ANCD Position Paper. Drug Testing*. ANCD (http://www.atoda.org.au/wp-content/uploads/DrugTesting2.pdf).

Ball J (2013) Silk Road: the online drug marketplace that officials seem powerless to stop. *The Guardian*, 22 March (http://www.theguardian.com/world/2013/mar/22/silk-road-online-drug-marketplace).

Blakemore SJ, Choudhury S (2006) Development of the adolescent brain: implications for executive function and social cognition. *Journal of Child Psychology and Psychiatry*, **47**, 296–312.

Borgelt LM, Franson KL, Nussbaum AM, *et al* (2013) The pharmacologic and clinical efects of medical cannabis. *Pharmacotherapy*, **33**, 195–209.

Crone EA, Dahl RA (2012) Understanding adolescence as a period of social–affective engagement and goal flexibility. *Nature Reviews Neuroscience*, **13**, 636–50.

Dargan PI, Tang HC, Liang W, *et al* (2014) Three months of methoxetamine administration is associated with significant bladder and renal toxicity in mice. *Clinical Toxicology (Philadelphia, Pa.)*, **52**, 176–80.

Department for Education (2013) *Personal, Social, Health and Economic (PSHE) Education*. Department for Education (https://www.gov.uk/government/publications/personal-social-health-and-economic-education-pshe/personal-social-health-and-economic-pshe-education).

Department of Health (2007) *Drug Misuse and Dependence: UK Guidelines on Clinical Management*. Department of Health (England), the Scottish Government, Welsh Assembly Government and Northern Ireland Executive

Di Forti M, Marconi A, Carra E, *et al* (2015) Proportion of patients in south London with first-episode psychosis attributable to use of high potency cannabis: a case-control study. *Lancet Psychiatry*, **2**, 233–8.

European Commission (2014) *Flash Eurobarometer 401: Young People and Drugs*. European Commission (http://ec.europa.eu/public_opinion/flash/fl_401_present_en.pdf).

European Monitoring Centre for Drugs and Drug Addiction (2014) *EMCDDA–Europol 2013 Annual Report on the Implementation of Council Decision 2005/387/JHA*. Publications Office of the European Union.

European Monitoring Centre for Drugs and Drug Addiction (2015) *New Psychoactive Substances in Europe: An Update from the EU Early Warning System*. European Monitoring Centre for Drugs and Drug Addiction.

Faggiano F, Monozzi S, Versino E, *et al* (2014) Universal school-based prevention for illicit drug use. *Cochrane Database Systematic Reviews*, **12**, CD003020.

General Medical Council (2007) *0–18 Years: Guidance for All Doctors*. GMC (http://www.gmc-uk.org/static/documents/content/0-18_years_-_English_1015.pdf).

Glantz MD, Anthony JC, Berglund PA, *et al* (2009) Mental disorders as risk factors for later substance dependence: estimates of optimal prevention and treatment benefits. *Psychological Medicine*, **39**, 1365–77.

Halpern JH, Pope HG Jr (2003) Hallucinogen persisting perception disorder: what do we know after 50 years? Drug and Alcohol Dependence, 69, 109–19.

Harris CR, Brown A (2013) Synthetic cannabinoid intoxication: a case series and review. *Journal of Emergency Medicine*, **44**, 360–6.

Health and Social Care Information Centre (2015) *Smoking, Drinking and Drug Use Among Young People in England in 2014*. National Statistics.

Home Office (2014) *Drug Misuse: Findings from the 2013/14 Crime Survey for England and Wales*. The Stationery Office.

Leeman RF, Potenza MN (2012) Similarities and differences between pathological gambling and substance use disorders: a focus on impulsivity and compulsivity. *Psychopharmacology*, **219**, 469–90.

Marmot M, Allen J, Goldblatt P, *et al* (2010) *Fair Society, Healthy Lives. The Marmot Review*. UCL Institute of Health Equity.

Manrique-Garcia E, Zammita S, Dalmana C, *et al* (2012) Cannabis, schizophrenia and other non-afective psychoses: 35 years of follow-up of a population-based cohort. *Psychological Medicine*, **42**, 1321–8.

McArdle P, Wiegersma A, Gilvarry E, *et al* (2002) European adolescent substance use: the roles of family structure, function and gender. *Addiction*, **97**, 329–36.

Measham F, Moore K, Østergaard J (2011) Mephedrone, 'Bubble' and unidentified white powders: the contested identities of synthetic 'legal highs'. *Drugs and Alcohol Today*, **11**, 137–146.

Mentor-ADEPIS (2014) *Quality Standards for Effective Alcohol and Drug Education*. Alcohol and Drug Education and Prevention Information Service.

Miech RA, Johnston LD, O'Malley PM, *et al* (2015) *Monitoring the Future: National Survey Results on Drug Use, 1975–2014. Volume 1, Secondary School Students*. The University of Michigan.

Moran PB, Vuchinich S, Hall NK (2004) Associations between types of maltreatment and substance use during adolescence. *Child Abuse and Neglect*, **28**, 529–39.

National Anthrax Outbreak Control Team (2011) *An Outbreak of Anthrax Among Drug Users in Scotland, December 2009 to December 2010*. Health Protection Scotland.

National Institute for Health and Care Excellence (2007*a*) *Interventions to Reduce Substance Misuse Among Vulnerable Young People* (Public Health Guidance 4). NICE.

National Institute for Health and Care Excellence (2007*b*) *Drug Misuse in Over 16s: Psychosocial Interventions* (CG51). NICE.

National Institute for Health and Care Excellence (2011) *Psychosis with Coexisting Substance Misuse: Assessment and Management in Adults and Young People* (CG120). NICE.

Nutt D, King LA, Saulbury W, *et al* (2007) Development of a rational scale to assess the harm of drugs of potential misuse. *Lancet*, **369**, 1047–53.

Nutt DJ, King LA, Phillips LD (2010) Drug harms in the UK: a multicriteria decision analysis. *The Lancet*, **376**, 1558–65.

Oetting ER, Beauvais F (1987) Peer cluster theory, socialization characteristics, and adolescent drug use: A path analysis. *Journal of Counseling Psychology*, **34**, 205–13.

Public Health England (2014) *Drug Treatment in England 2013–14*. PHE.

Public Health England (2015) *Substance Misuse Among Young People in England 2013–14*. PHE.

Realini N, Rubino T, Parolaro D (2009) Neurobiological alterations at adult age triggered by adolescent exposure to cannabinoids. *Pharmacological Research*, **60**, 132–8.

Royal Society for the Encouragement of Arts, Manufactures and Commerce (2007) *Drugs – Facing Facts*. RSA.

Shulgin A, Shulgin A (1991) *PIHKAL: A Chemical Love Story*. Transform Press.

Staiger PK, Kambouropoulos N, Dawe S (2007) Should personality traits be considered when refining substance misuse treatment programmes? *Drug and Alcohol Review*, **26**, 17–23.

Steinberg L (2008) A social neuroscience perspective on adolescent risk-taking. *Developmental Review*, **28**, 78–106.

Swendsen J, Le Moal M (2011) individual vulnerability to addiction. *Annals of the New York Academy of Sciences*, **1216**, 73–85.

Taylor R (2015) Ross Ulbricht: Silk Road creator convicted on drugs charges. *BBC News*, 2 February (http://www.bbc.co.uk/news/world-us-canada-31134938).

The Psychologist (2015) Teenagers debunked [transcript]. *The Psychologist* (https://thepsychologist.bps.org.uk/teenagers-debunked).

Tsuang MT, Lyons MJ, Meyer JM, *et al* (1998) Co-occurrence of abuse of different drugs in men: the role of drug-specific and shared vulnerabilities. *Archives of General Psychiatry*, **55**, 967–72.

United Nations Office on Drugs and Crime (2013) *The Challenge of New Psychoactive Substances*. United Nations.

United Nations Office on Drugs and Crime (2014) *World Drug Report 2014*. United Nations.

Winstock AR, Griffiths P, Stewart D (2001) Drugs and the dance music scene: a survey of current drug use patterns among a sample of dance music enthusiasts in the UK. *Drug and Alcohol Dependence*, **64**, 9–17.

Winstock AR, Barratt MJ (2013) Synthetic cannabis: a comparison of patterns of use and effect profile with natural cannabis in a large global sample. *Drug and Alcohol Dependence*, **131**, 106–11.

World Health Organization (2009) *Interpersonal Violence and Illicit Drugs*. WHO.

World Health Organization (2014) *Global Status Report on Alcohol and Health 2014*. WHO.

World Health Organization (2015a) *Management of Substance Abuse: Harmful Use*. WHO (http://www.who.int/substance_abuse/terminology/definition2/en).

World Health Organization (2015b) *Management of Substance Abuse: Dependence Syndrome*. WHO (http://www.who.int/substance_abuse/terminology/definition1/en).

Index